Baby Boomers' Me

MW01714926

MAKING YOUR OWN CHOICES

Through the Other End of Puberty

CAROLYN AGOSTA

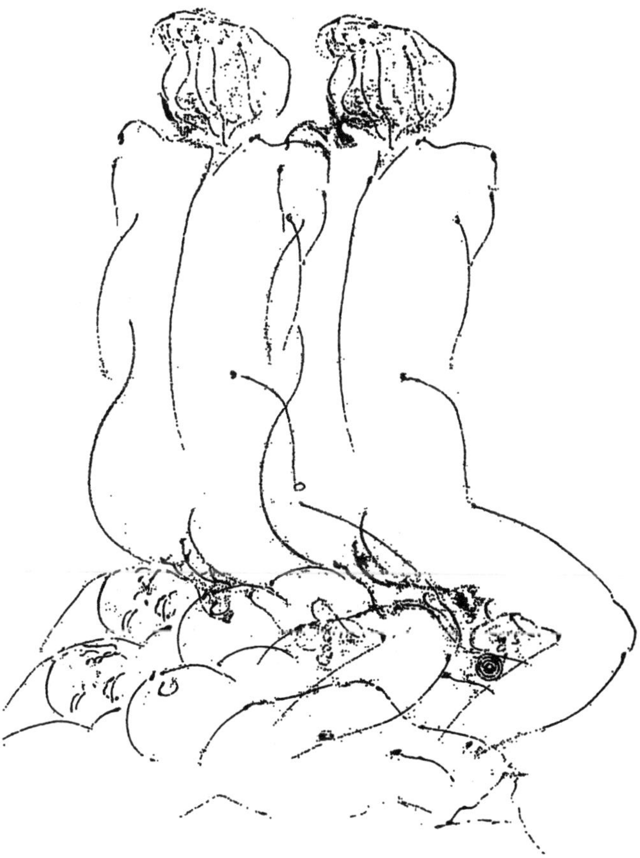

CA PUBLISHING, INK

Printed and Bound in the United States of America

Distributed in the United States by CA Publishing, Ink

Gualala, California

Cover Layout and Design by Gale Mettey

Artwork by Willa Marten

Permission for quotes from Rebecca Latimer's book *You're Not Old Until You're Ninety* was graciously granted by Paul M. Clemens, Publisher, Blue Dolphin Publishing, Inc.

CA Publishing, Ink

35501 South Highway One, Unit 103

Gualala, CA 95445-5103

To purchase copies of this book, contact CA Publishing at menopausebook.org or send check or money order for $12.95 plus $2.00 postage and handling to: CA Publishing, 35501 South Highway One, Unit 103, Gualala, CA 95445-5103. Allow three weeks for delivery. (See Order Form page 66)

International Standards Book Number: 0-9702293-0-5

Dedicated to my mother,

Veronica,

who raised eight kids

in a time of major transition

for women

and who helped to make me

the woman

I am today.

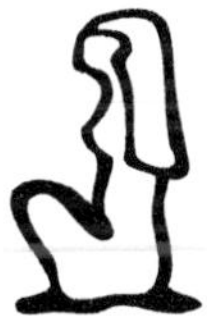

Acknowledgments

Special thanks to my husband, Terry Albertson, for all of his emotional, physical, spiritual, and financial support. Thanks also to Dr. Deborah Flick and Kelly White for their gentle readership. Thank you tons and bunches to Dr. Gary Klepper and Dr. Sumedha Khanna for their editing suggestions and encouragement. My women's writing group was a special source of encouragement and support. Also, thank you to Sheldon Gerstein, Editor and Publisher of *Coast Magazine* in Northern California for his support, encouragement, and derriere kicking through a difficult time. A huge thank you to Drs. Lois Johnson (medical doctor) and Gary Klepper (holistic doctor) for their guidance through my menopause. An enormous thank you to Judy Hooper, Ph.D. and Roberta Jones, for their wonderful editing and proofing talents. Their eagle eyes and knowledge of the English language were invaluable! A special thanks to the women interviewed for their frankness in discussing the topic.

Tons of thanks to my mother, brother, Paul, and sister, Kate for their belief in me and willingness to back that faith financially!

And last, but not least, to Willa Marten for her spectacular art work and to Gale Mettey for the time and creative juices she used to make this book gorgeous. Thank you so much!

Table of Contents ~

What Is HRT?

CHAPTER SIX

pages 29–35

Alternatives to HRT

CHAPTER SEVEN

pages 37–53

Summary

CHAPTER EIGHT

pages 55–56

For More Information

CHAPTER NINE

pages 57–60

Glossary of Common Terms

CHAPTER TEN

pages 61–64

We always attract into our lives whatever we think about most, believe in most strongly, expect on the deepest level, and imagine most vividly.

Shakti Gawain

~ Introduction ~

A close friend urged me to use this introduction to tell people about myself. She said, "They need to understand where you've been and why you are the best person to write this book. Tell them about yourself, the real you. Tell them so they know why it's logical that you are writing this book, and that it's worth reading." So here goes ...

At the age of eighteen, I was your average young woman from an Italian, Catholic family. Shy, quiet, traditional, reserved, a college student, plugging along, working on my MRS. (as we used to joke), a child of the early 60s, bound for change.

At the age of twenty, I went to visit my pregnant girlfriend and her husband, where I managed to secure a waitressing job fairly easily. Two days later, I was a rape statistic. On a date with a fellow employee, I fought to prevent it, and lost. A part of me died that day. But as the third of eight children in a family of activists, I was destined to recover.

I went from feeling dead inside to anger and rage about everything: sexism, racism, the war, and the lack of choices for women. Every week I was demonstrating, shouting, screaming my outrage at the injustices in the world. In 1969, I quit my job to drive with friends to Washington, DC and work with the Vietnam Veterans Against the War. Then in 1973, frustrated with the movements, I moved to Denver, returned to college, earning a Bachelor of Science in Human Services with a minor in Psychology. I took all of the women's studies courses that were available (not many at the time). I had decided that if I couldn't change the world by demonstrating, I'd change it by helping people heal. A year after receiving my BS, I went on to earn my Master's degree in Social Work.

On the side, studying self-defense and home security, I learned what women needed to change our attitudes. I developed a self-defense program for women, altruistically believing that I could teach every Denver woman to protect herself from rape. For seven years, the Denver Police Department sponsored it. After reading every book published on rape at the time and studying therapeutic interventions, a friend and I developed a treatment program for rape victims and set-up a support group for women, so every victim in Denver could heal. (This was prior to the time that I learned that men could be victims too.) The local mental health center sponsored and provided clinical supervision for the group. Denver didn't have a hotline for victims at the time; my home phone became the hotline. Calls came in the middle of the night. I'd meet the victim at her home, usually arriving before the police. Sometimes, many times, the women hadn't even called the police yet. Sure it felt crazy, a little scary, *and* I wanted to make a difference.

Right out of graduate school, I was hired as the Program Director of Denver SafeHouse for Battered Women, the only long-term shelter in the country at the time. I continued teaching self-defense classes, trained new instructors, set up the Self-Protection Instruction Team (SPIT), and continued offering a support group for rape victims. On weekends and evenings, I provided training to professionals, other therapists, police officers, and medical doctors, on the treatment of rape victims. Traveling all over the country, I taught workshops, spoke at conferences, and provided in-service training. My life became my work ... and my work became my life. As long as women were being raped, I could not rest.

The Executive Director of SafeHouse resigned and in 1978 the board hired me as director. At the time federal funds for victims of crime were available. In 1980, all of the three-year grants ended and everyone was scrambling for money. My job became less about serving people and more about fund-raising. Not what I wanted. Another woman (also a former rape victim) and I founded our own program, EVE, Ending Violence Effectively, Inc. With my experience and reputation, women were referred to us by every agency in the city. Four months after opening our doors, we held our first open house. It was attended by the mayor, Representative Pat Schroeder, the Denver DA, most of the directors of the local mental health centers, many top-ranking police officers, and dozens of family and friends. Just getting all those folks in the same room made us believe we were on our way to making a real difference!

With Colorado Outward Bound School, we developed the first wilderness therapy program. It received international notoriety. Mental health centers and police departments both locally and nationally requested training from us, made referrals to our program, and asked for consultation. We were invited to speak at every statewide mental health conference from 1975 to 1988. Through it all, my goal was to change the lives of victims of rape and incest, and battered women, helping them take their awful, horrible, painful experience and use it to learn — coming out the other end a stronger, healthier person. I worked to change the laws, making it easier for a victim to come forward and speak the truth. It was important to me that other women had more support than I did when I was a victim.

Laws changed. Programs developed. Now almost every street corner in any major city has an expert in the treatment of victims and there is a victim compensation program in most counties throughout the US. After twenty years of giving my heart and soul, I knew it was time to move on. I handed EVE over to my business partner, Mary, and left Colorado.

In 1992, with my husband, I moved to a small community in Northern California where I was hired by a local magazine to sell ads and write articles. I'd written technical articles about rape, incest, and battered women; written passionate articles about the impact of trauma on victims and their families, but this was a whole new ball game. I interviewed artists, wrote fiction and non-fiction articles. I loved it! Life was calm, peaceful. Lunches were on the office deck, looking at the ocean. No presentations, no gobbled lunches while driving, no dinner meetings, no breakfast meetings, no lunch meetings!

It was while sitting in this peaceful environment that I received a call from my doctor about the results of my blood tests. She began asking me questions about possible symptoms related to menopause. My estrogen level was low and I had major symptoms of perimenopause. (I didn't even know what the word meant at the time!) I was glad to be alone in the office, because I began to cry. I thought menopause happened to really old women; I was young, only forty-five.

I wonder if I'd never received that call, would my symptoms have been less pronounced? Would I have been able to ignore the changes in my body? I wonder if it weren't thrown in our faces as such an ugly, dehumanizing experience, would we respond differently? I don't have the answer. We live in a society that believes "old" is over thirty-nine. Perhaps we "baby boomers" can change that image.

My doctor wanted me to start on hormone replacement therapy immediately. I tried arguing with her, "Don't all women go through this? We can't all need to take pills!" She argued back, "Yes all women go through this, and for their own health, they'd better go on hormone replacement therapy (HRT)." I hated the idea of taking drugs. Never having been a person to accept what I am told as gospel, I wanted to know why. She told me that HRT reduces the risk of heart attack, prevents osteoporosis, and makes you feel young. I wasn't buying it. Through my tears, I explained, "I take calcium and magnesium every day, eat calcium-rich foods, exercise almost daily, eat a low fat, high fiber diet. So won't that protect me?" "Not as much as HRT," she argued. Her message was strong, compelling, and she was, after all, a medical doctor.

"But I'm high risk for breast cancer, shouldn't I avoid HRT?" Here was her critical mistake. She said, "If you get breast cancer, we can cure it. If you have a heart attack and die, there's nothing we can do." Having just buried a friend, a young woman who'd died from breast cancer, I knew she was wrong. Quietly, the tears still streaming down my face, I said, "I'll think about it," and hung up the phone.

Once again, I was ready for a fight! I called a holistic doctor and scheduled an appointment, began my search for a new medical doctor, and ordered several books on menopause. When I told my editor, Sheldon, about the conversation, he urged me to write about it. That began serious research on the subject of menopause — research that would continue for the next several years, resulting in changing my life (again) and a series of articles that would get the coast of northern California buzzing.

It amazes me that it took me forty-five years to learn about my own body! The good news is that I know so much more and am continuing to learn. My friends jokingly refer to me as "Doctor" Agosta. Let me make this very clear, I am not a doctor. I am a woman, a fighter, a person who is always determined to make life better for me and for anyone with whom I come in contact.

My goal in writing this book, like my goal in working with victims of violence, is to use what I have learned to help women take a new experience and learn from it — coming out the other end a stronger, healthier, happier person. ▣

How to use this book~

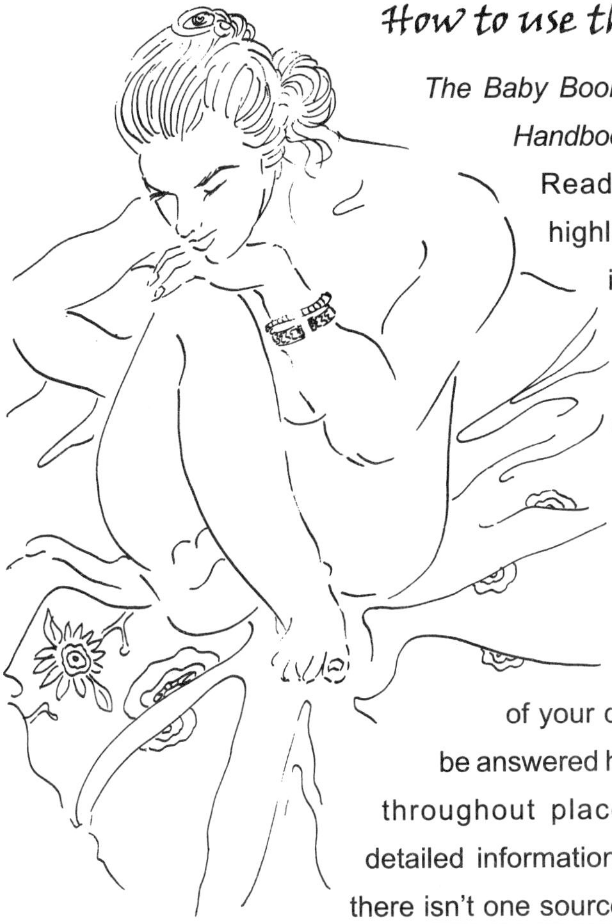

The Baby Boomers' Menopause Handbook is user friendly. Read it through and highlight the areas of importance to you. If there are words or terms that you do not understand, definitions are in the glossary in Chapter 10. This is a guidebook; consequently, all of your questions may not be answered here. I've indicated throughout places to find more detailed information. Remember that there isn't one source that can answer all you want to know about your body.

This book is a resource to help you access information and to help simplify some of the information that is available. It is a combination of my research and the experiences of many other women. There are places that will touch you personally and speak to you. Use what is valuable to you. Leave the rest. After all, only you know what is best for you. Trust your own instincts and read all you can in order to educate yourself. Good luck! I'm on your side!

My only advice is to stay aware, listen carefully, and yell for help if you need it.

Judy Blume

CHAPTER ONE:
Other Women's Experiences

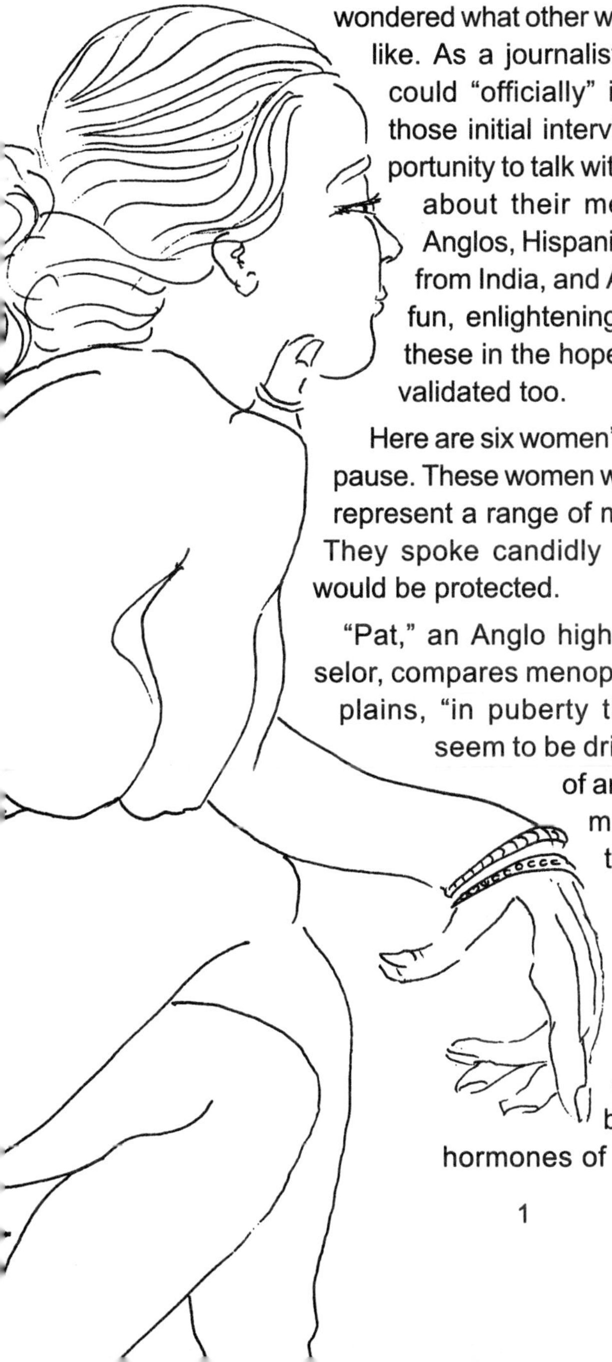

As I began thinking about my own menopause, I wondered what other women's experiences were like. As a journalist for a local magazine, I could "officially" interview women. Since those initial interviews, I have had the opportunity to talk with dozens of other women about their menopause experiences: Anglos, Hispanics, Black women, women from India, and Asian women. It has been fun, enlightening, and validating. I share these in the hopes that you learn and feel validated too.

Here are six women's experiences with menopause. These women were chosen because they represent a range of menopausal experiences. They spoke candidly knowing their identities would be protected.

"Pat," an Anglo high school guidance counselor, compares menopause to puberty. She explains, "in puberty the floor falls out. Girls seem to be driven wild, crazy, with lots of anger, while boys flex their muscles developing a tough guy attitude. Menopause is the opposite of that." Gail Sheehy in *The Silent Passage* reinforces that idea, "The raging hormones of adolescence suddenly become the unraging hormones of menopause."

"Sheree"

Sheree is a Black woman and a real estate agent. Her experience with menopause was almost non-existent. "I don't think I had 'hot flashes.' I just noticed at one time that I didn't need to wear as many clothes and didn't get cold as easily as I used to. That's about it." Having spoken with her mother about menopause, her mother laughed telling her they didn't have time for such luxuries.

Neither she nor her sister ever went to a doctor for treatment of menopausal symptoms, nor did they ever consider hormone replacement. She reports that her periods became "a little weird, you know, more frequent, less frequent, heavier, lighter, that sort of thing." Other than noticing the changes, she never felt compelled to do anything about them. After six months of no periods, she thought, "Thank God that's over," and happily gave her remaining pads and tampons to her younger sister. "It was no big deal and I don't know what all the fuss is about. It was a whole lot easier than puberty, which was hell!—mostly because my hormones were kicking in and I was crazy about the boys. I highly recommend menopause—no periods, no birth control. It's great!"

"Billie"

Billie, an Anglo woman and a masseuse, has a different story to share. Her first indications of menopause were shifts in her menstrual cycle during her late 30s. Her cycle went from twenty-eight days to nineteen. At about age forty-two, her doctor attributed a change in her nervous system to menopause. The change caused dry mouth and nasal passages to dilate when they shouldn't. Suddenly she developed allergies and sinus problems. "I'm confused about what symptoms to attach to hormone level shifts. There is so much the literature hasn't covered." At age forty-six, she finds herself much more sensitive to chemicals, pollen, "everything," things to which she'd never reacted.

Periodically she finds herself dropping "into a hole" in which she personalizes "everything." For a brief period of time, she had several panic attacks. "My heart was racing, I thought I'd die." Rushing to medical treatment, she was given a shot of cortisone and anti-biotics. A few days later, she had a second "full-blown" attack. Again, rushing to medical treatment, she received Xanax, a highly addictive anti-depressant. She took this for several days, then decided to stop using it. She experienced several smaller attacks within a few days of each other. She has had none since.

Billie has become very sensitive to touch. When her partner touches her now, "it goes deep inside" and at times she is brought to tears by it. She wishes men could understand the tenderness and need for gentle touch, even more than the act of intercourse.

She doesn't expect to take hormones, "besides if nature wanted us to have estrogen, we would. I've just become more conscious of my eating habits. Diet can help a lot." Thin bones cause her concern about osteoporosis. She takes vitamins, including 500 mg. of calcium, eats lots of fruits and vegetables, very little dairy, and pays attention to the effect different foods have on her, trying to eat intelligently. She attends aerobics classes several times a week and takes walks daily. She began Jin Shin Jyutsu treatments over a year ago and has found them to be tremendously helpful in feeling balanced.

Recently, Billie's life has become even more stressful. Her mood swings have been extreme, at times, debilitating. She vacillates between trying to regulate herself and emergency room treatment when she hits "rock bottom." She continues to struggle with menopausal symptoms.

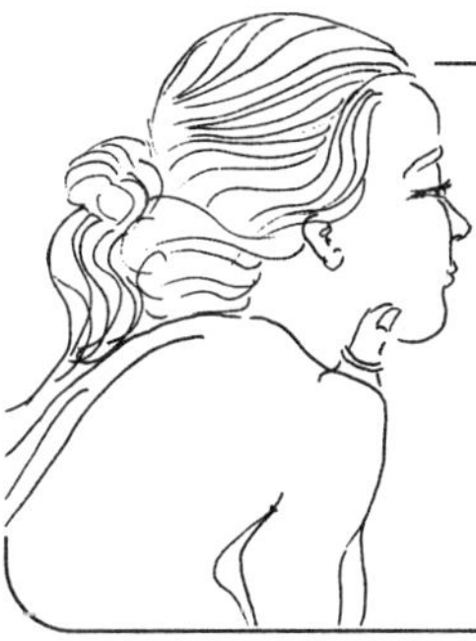

The history of all times, and of today especially, teaches that ... women will be forgotten if they forget to think about themselves.

Louise Otto

"Esther"

Fifty-three year old Esther officially began menopause in her mid-40s. Reflecting on memories of her mother in menopause — hot flashes and violent mood swings, Esther suspects her mother felt very alone since she had no women friends. Esther explains that the male members of the family had only contempt for their mother, disgustedly commenting, "Oh, there goes mom again."

Esther, an Anglo woman and struggling artist, explains that her menopause experiences have been wrought with fear and pain. She attributes it, in part, to her younger years. In her 20s, she took a 5 mg. estrogen/progesterone birth control pill daily until, at thirty, she had a stroke. Her temporary paralysis terrified her. Between birth control pills and blood pressure medicine she felt like a guinea pig. With this background, she wondered what shape her system was in entering menopause.

In her mid-30s, she had a tubal ligation causing symptoms of perimenopause. "My blood pressure shot up. I became depressed. I had hot flashes all the time and severe panic attacks causing me to seek medical help regularly. But no connection was ever made between menopause and my attacks. My attacks became so severe that I couldn't continue working. I quit my job and moved." When a therapist told her that she was having panic attacks, she was relieved. Once she knew what they were, she was able to control them. She found that jogging or breathing into a paper bag calmed her. On one trip to the emergency room, she was given Xanax. "I pop one on rare occasions, when it happens at night." Now the panic attacks are infrequent.

Her doctor reported finding nothing in the literature about the connection between the adrenals, nervous system, and hormones. There was little about menopause in the early 80s. Recently, while reading *Women of the Thirteenth Moon*, she "found herself" in one of the articles. A woman wrote about her menopause experience; it was identical to Esther's. Suddenly, she felt "normal."

Esther has been on HRT (hormonal replacement therapy) for

ten years. When she began, it was "like coming out of a tunnel." She takes one estrogen pill the first day, two the next, alternating each day; on days 16–25 she adds progestin. Each time she sees her doctor, she asks how much longer she will be on them. Concerned that Esther's periods have continued, her doctor hesitates to guess. Esther's menstrual cycle had stopped for nine months, now she is back to normal periods. "The alternative to HRT is so awful, but I'm afraid I'll have periods the rest of my life!"

She is angry that Western medicine is not looking into alternatives, using herbs and Eastern medicine. She says that she won't take herbs, they are too experimental, yet she feels Western medicine has been experimenting on her all of her life. Esther does take vitamins, in particular, oyster calcium, about 600 mg. per day and she walks daily. Meditating has helped her to feel grounded.

Esther finally confronted her doctor with the risk factors of being treated with HRT long term; consequently, her doctor lowered her dose. Esther is afraid to disagree with her doctor, so she remains on HRT.

"Pat"

Menopause for Pat, a fifty-year-old Anglo woman and therapist, began in 1992. She was furious with her mother, " Why didn't you tell me? Why didn't you warn me? You should've told me!" But her mother's generation was taught never to discuss it. "Our mothers pretended that they weren't going through it—it meant getting old. This is the perfect time to go through menopause. So many women

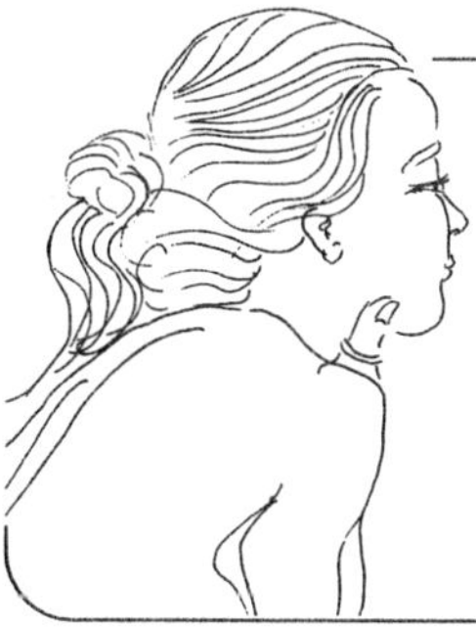

> Bit by bit...she had claimed herself. Freeing yourself was one thing; claiming ownership of that freed self was another.
>
> *Toni Morrison*

are going through it now. We're talking about it. I don't feel alone." Identical to her mother's experience, Pat's periods were gradually closer together with heavier flows, then further apart, lighter and shorter. Pat has not had a period since 1994.

She had numerous panic attacks — "free-floating anxiety attacks. It's like an unknown force enters your body. I don't feel grounded, not on my two feet. Things trigger them that never would have before. I take a normal event and blow it out of proportion." Including dry mouth, heart beating fast, feeling out of control, they continue on and off for two or three days. "I needed to get clinical about it saying 'this will pass.'" She had them for two years; then they diminished. Now they are gone.

Her memory and coordination were affected; she regularly drops and breaks glasses and bowls. Her arms feel weak. She also finds that she is very sensitive to touch. "It has to be firm. Especially during sex, I like a lot of touch even though my breasts are often tender."

The most annoying experience was hot flashes. She would have five or six a night, leaving her exhausted and sleep deprived. She'd feel too hot and throw the covers off, then become chilled and pull them back on. Lack of sleep is what led her to hormone replacement therapy. She says, "Without estrogen, that sense of well-being is gone."

She was prescribed Premarin® (synthetic estrogen replacement) daily and 10 mg. of progestin (progesterone replacement) 10 days of the month. "It just didn't make sense to me, I could never do it, not even for a month." She learned that a doctor in southern California recommended low doses of estrogen daily and progestin (2.5 mg.) only ten days of every three months. "So I cut both pills in half, took the Premarin® daily and the progestin three or four days of the month. You know your own body and have to trust yourself. The prescriptions are so standard for everyone, you just have to know what is best for you." Now she takes estrogen when she feels she needs it, every once in a while. She reports that it works for her.

Almost through menopause, she feels more confident and comfortable in her work than ever before. She finds she has less need for approval or to compete. She takes walks regularly, is trying to eat more healthy foods, and recently added a lightweight workout to her regime.

"Ruby"

A fifty-three-year-old Native American post-menopausal woman, Ruby's experience with perimenopause was minimal. At forty-nine, she missed one period. They had always been very short, two days. At fifty, a pattern of missed periods developed, every two or three months. At fifty-one her periods stopped and never continued again.

Her only discomfort was at the time her periods were scheduled to occur; she experienced mild premenstrual syndrome (PMS.) Ruby never noticed any emotional responses to diminished hormones.

When asked if she'd noticed any change since menopause, she talked about relationships, in particular intimate ones. She no longer wants "a partner just for the sake of sex." She wants more closeness, more connection with another person, a life-mate with similar spiritual awareness, as she says, "reaching the spiritual through the sexual."

She attributes her ease through the pause as a result of several factors. She doesn't accept white cultural biases about women and believes she has more control of her life and her body. In addition, she eats a low fat, mainly vegetarian diet, doesn't drink alcohol or

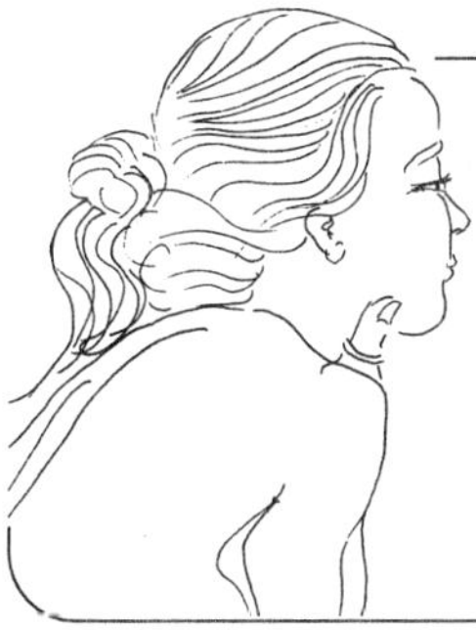

The being cannot be termed rational or virtuous, who obeys any authority, but that of reason.

Mary Wollenstonecraft

smoke cigarettes, takes a combination of vitamins and herbs, and she exercises two or three times a week, including yoga and dance. In the past year, Ruby has begun using a wild yam cream and GLA (see Chapter 8 for more information) as part of her post-menopausal routine.

"Sarah"

At forty-six, Sarah, an Anglo shop owner, knew she was going through the pause, she just didn't know what it meant. Her periods began to change in her late 30s. Then they became unpredictable, every two weeks for a while, lasting three days, then nothing for six weeks followed by a heavy flow lasting a week or two or even three.

"My first panic attack really frightened me. I thought I was going to die. It came suddenly, just a reaction to a minor event and I was off. My heart was pounding so hard, I thought it would explode out of my rib cage. I couldn't slow it down and I couldn't catch my breath." She cried, tried to regain her "composure" and finally went for a long rigorous walk. "That helped. Out in the wilderness, I screamed and cried to my heart's content." At the time she didn't know what was happening. After talking to several other menopausal friends, she was relieved to learn that her panic attack was part of menopause — she wasn't going crazy!

"You can't imagine what it's like to suddenly lose control of yourself, feeling like a crazy woman. Now that I know what it is, I'm better equipped to handle it. If there is a next time, I know it will pass. Get away from people, walk, and breathe deeply."

Her hot flashes were different than what she had read, heard or expected. "I don't sweat a lot, but then I'm not a big sweater anyway. Heat begins in my gut and spreads through my entire body, there's a brief feeling of weakness and it passes. At the most, it lasts several minutes." She had hot flashes at night and like so many other women, spent the night removing and replacing covers, not sleeping as soundly as she once did. She says she just accepted it. "I just get up and write or read, then go back to bed when I feel sleepy. I actually enjoy the time alone."

Exercising five or six times a week including light weights helps her feel good. She's eaten a low fat diet free of animal products for fifteen years and takes vitamins and minerals with the guidance of a holistic doctor. "As far as I can tell, my body decided it's time to stop producing hormones, so I'll deal with heart disease and osteoporosis by maintaining good health. Period."

Now postmenopause, Sarah never took hormones and kept to her regimen. She still uses a wild yam cream, vitamin E, and GLA from evening primrose oil or borage oil, and a tincture of black cohosh to help her. Two years postmenopause, she has occasional "warm flushes," and is not bothered by any other symptoms.

Summary

Most of the women interviewed wished they could take time alone for a few months without interference, to evaluate the first half of their lives and plan for the second. (It seems that women and men could benefit from time alone at this point in their lives.)

Sex can often be a difficult subject; these women discussed it with ease. Two of the women noticed a considerable drop in their sex drive and accepted it. One hoped she'd recover her "lost" libido, sometime. The other three women found themselves becoming more comfortable sexually. Orgasms had become less intense or less frequent. One woman described it as a "sweetness" about sex without the urgency of youth.

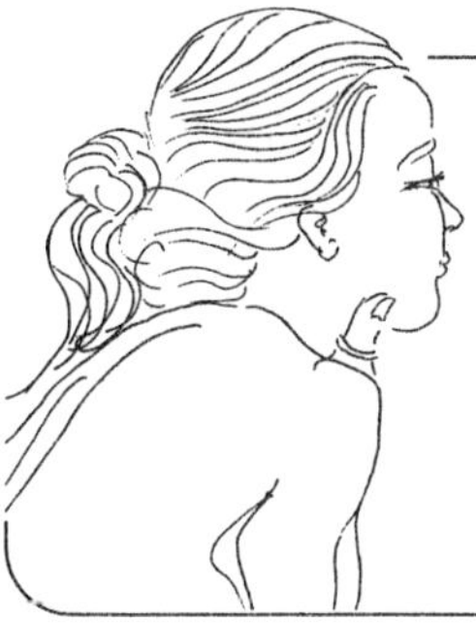

Nothing in life is to be feared.
It is only to be understood.

Marie Curie

I feel there is something unexplored about woman that only woman can explore.

Georgia O'Keeffe

CHAPTER TWO:
What Is Menopause?

The word menopause is borrowed from the Greeks: "meno" meaning month when used with "pause" to form the word "menopause." The Cambridge Encyclopedia 1992 edition says: "Menopause is unique to the human female, but its significance is unclear." Therein lies the problem.

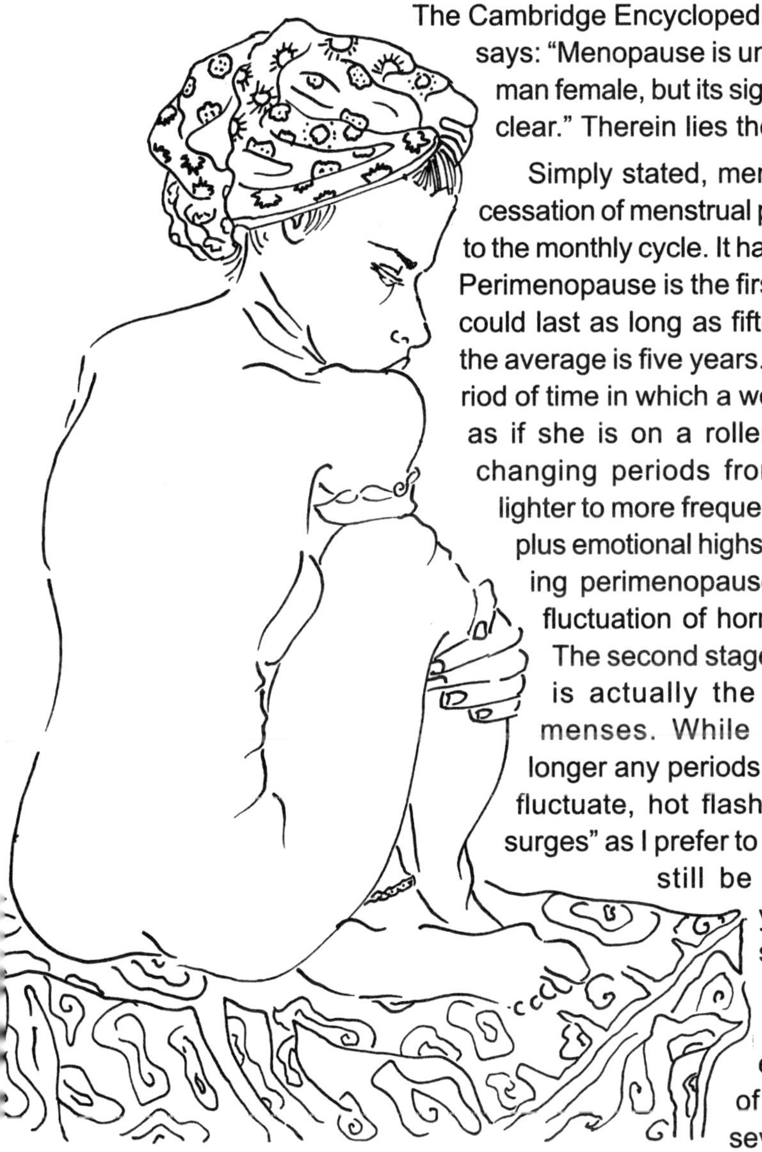

Simply stated, menopause is the cessation of menstrual periods, an end to the monthly cycle. It has three stages. Perimenopause is the first stage, which could last as long as fifteen years, but the average is five years. This is the period of time in which a woman may feel as if she is on a roller coaster with changing periods from longer and lighter to more frequent and heavier, plus emotional highs and lows. During perimenopause the greatest fluctuation of hormones occurs. The second stage, menopause, is actually the cessation of menses. While there are no longer any periods, emotions can fluctuate, hot flashes (or "power surges" as I prefer to call them) may still be present, and your body is still adjusting to the change in hormone levels. This period of time can last several years.

The final stage, which lasts the remainder of a woman's life, is postmenopause, the point at which you and your body are generally comfortable with your hormone level. During this last period of time, fluctuation in hormone levels may occur when foods containing hormones are added to the diet. (We'll discuss more on that in Chapter 7.)

Thirty, twenty, even ten years ago, menopause was rarely discussed. The babyboom generation has grown up with the women's movement; consequently, women are sharing more intimately with each other, discussing what is happening to their bodies, and replacing negative stereotypes. Menopause is a phase in a woman's life—and, as with all phases of human life, sometimes one needs help with it and sometimes not. In the *Harvard Women's Health Watch*, August 1998, they state, "In some ways, menopause is similar to pregnancy. It is a natural, healthy state that nonetheless may require some attention."

Menopause is a time of change: physical, emotional, psychological, spiritual. Change. Not necessarily unpleasant, perhaps unexpected. No matter how positive, change is difficult. And the potential result? The obvious one is no more periods, but women say there is so much more. Women, aging like fine wine, improving with each year, throwing away stereotypes. Finally taking time for themselves, discovering who they are.

Right now the number of American women experiencing some form of menopause is forty-three million! (*The Silent Passage*) That's a relief because with those numbers, the experience must be normal.

Hormones at Work

The hormones (estrogen, progesterone, androgens, and many others) produced throughout a woman's life affect her general health and well being, including bone strength, sexuality, and reproduction. Understanding how these hormones affect a woman's cycle will help one to understand menopause.

During the first half of the menstrual cycle, the ovaries produce estrogen, which causes a thick lining to grow inside the uterus. At mid-cycle, one ovary releases an egg cell that travels down the

Fallopian tube into the uterus. (This is the time when pregnancy is most likely to occur.) During the next two weeks the ovary produces progesterone to strengthen the lining of the uterus and prepare for the fertile egg. If the egg is not fertilized, the levels of estrogen and progesterone diminish quickly; the lining of the uterus loses hormonal support and is shed during menstruation. Then the cycle begins again.

Estrogen protects arteries, increases production of HDLs (the "good" cholesterol) and reduces LDLs (the "bad" cholesterol), helps maintain bone mass by assisting calcium absorption, supports production of collagen (which maintains elasticity of the skin), and may protect against Alzheimer's disease.

Progesterone, produced by the ovaries and adrenals, has a calming effect on a woman, maintains the nervous system, and is the stimulator for new bone production. The lack of this hormone may be associated with mood swings, weight gain, anger and anxiety, depression, night sweats, osteoporosis, and diminished libido.

The hormone DHEA has received more attention in recent years. Produced mainly by the adrenal glands, it is associated with strengthening the immune system, reducing fat deposits in the arteries, improving cognition and mood, and promoting bone growth.

Androgens maintain strength, sex drive, and the elasticity of the vagina, as well as influencing general health. Some androgens are converted to estrogen in the fat cells of a woman's body. Recent

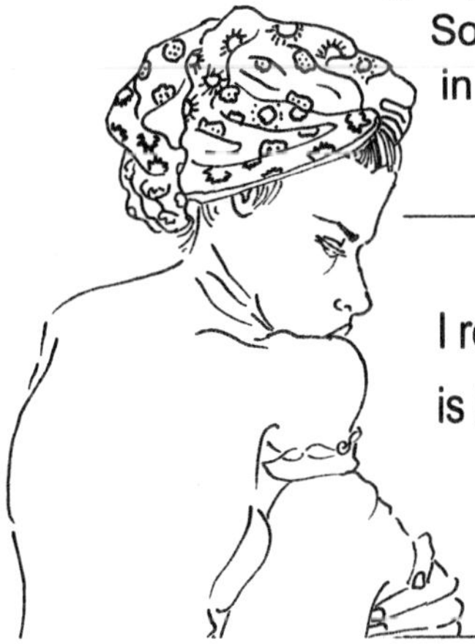

I restore myself when I'm alone. A career is born in public – talent in private.

Marilyn Monroe

studies indicate that even eighty-year-old women produce some androgens. Good reason to think twice about having healthy ovaries removed during a hysterectomy.

During perimenopause, which usually begins after forty (and sometimes earlier), your body runs out of eggs. Without eggs, there is little need for progesterone to strengthen the uterine lining. We still have periods. Your body continues to do what it's become accustomed to doing; it feels as if you are going to ovulate, then you don't.

What Menopause Is and Is Not

Menopause is not a disease. It is a normal part of the life cycle for all women. It is the body adjusting to changing hormones, a 40% decrease in estrogen and a drop to almost zero in progesterone. Other hormones diminish dramatically in varying degrees. As mentioned earlier, it is very much like the symptoms of puberty. Dr. Susan Love, explains in her book, *The Hormone Book:* "A study done in 1965 found that, with the exception of hot flashes, the symptoms of perimenopause were closer to those of adolescents entering puberty...When adolescent girls experience weight gain, bloating, and mood changes, doctors assume it's because of high estrogen levels. When women around menopause get the same symptoms, the assumption is that it's caused by low estrogen ... the time right before menopause is the mirror image of puberty. During puberty, this mechanism is starting up. Then, at the other end, when the process is gearing down, the same things happen again. What these two life stages have in common is big hormonal shifts. Times of hormonal shifts and changes are times of ... highs and lows ... you didn't know what was going on with your body...Well, with perimenopause it happens all over again ... Fortunately, *just as with puberty, these symptoms do end.*" (Emphasis mine.)

Gail Sheehy describes the menopausal years as the "time to render normalcy to a normal physical process that ushers in the youth of our Second Adulthood." She describes it as "a passage as momentous as the rite of passage into adolescence.

"Researchers now admit that they have underestimated the

number of younger women who experience symptoms of menopause even though they still have periods," explains Sheehy. We now know women as young as their late 30s begin experiencing changes in their menstrual cycle. These are early indicators of perimenopause.

Images of Menopause

The media has given us one image of menopause, that of an aging, dried up, miserable grouch. But there are many wonderful ways of viewing menopause: a metamorphosis, a time of complete change from one person to another (Weed), a time to find a new source of aliveness and meaning that will make the years ahead even more precious than those past. (Sheehy) If we understand the parallels between puberty and menopause, the whole thing is less scary and strange; we survived puberty, we'll survive menopause. (Love)

Joanna Baird Mallouk, RN and qualified homeopath Homotoxicologist adds, "Women have rights of passage for puberty, childbirth, menopause, and death. What is all the fuss about menopause? It is a natural phenomenon. Your body has enough estrogen to carry you from birth to death. At puberty and during your childbearing years, you have more. As you age, it diminishes because you don't need as much. It's a lot of hogwash when they give all women extra estrogen. It only creates more problems for the body." Many of her clients in Toronto are menopausal women whom she has helped using herbs and homeopathic remedies.

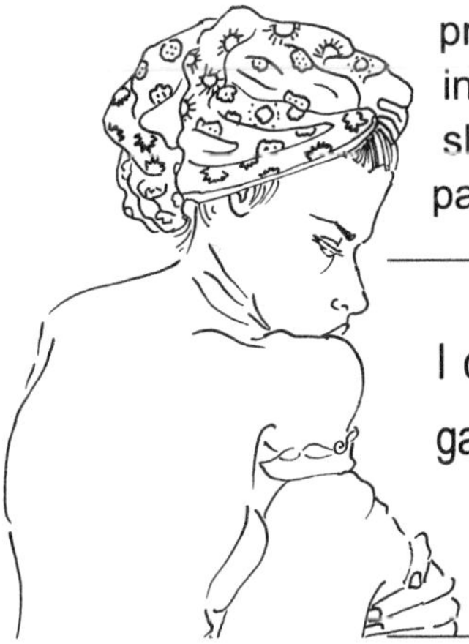

I contribute my success to this. I never gave or took an excuse.

Florence Nightingale

We are volcanoes. When we offer women our experience as our truth, as human truth, all the maps change. There are new mountains.

Ursula K. LeGuin

CHAPTER THREE:

Not All Estrogens Are Created Equal

Most of us think that estrogen is estrogen. In fact, there are three types of estrogen in a woman's body: estrone (E1), estradiol (E2), and estriol (E3). Estradiol is produced directly by the ovaries. Estrone is formed from the conversion of estradiol. Estriol, a somewhat weaker estrogen, is also produced in much smaller amounts by the ovaries. Estrone and estradiol are used in conventional hormone replacement therapy and are the estrogens associated with breast cancer. Estriol (E3) has a protective effect against breast and uterine cancer. A healthy liver converts estrone (E1) to estriol (E3). A diminished Estrogen Quotient (EQ) is an indicator of a problem with liver detoxification. The human female reproductive system operates on these three separate estrogens: estriol, estradiol, and estrone, which occur in an approximate ratio of 90:7:3 percent.

Dr. Henry Lemon's research (1966, 1975, and 1980) strongly suggests that estriol is a breast cancer inhibitor. He (and others) claims that because it is a weak estrogen, it can be used in higher doses without risk to the user. Remission or arrest of cancer was noted in 37% of the breast cancer patients in one of his studies. The current treatment for breast cancer includes administering a drug known as Tamoxifen, which blocks the effects of estrone and estradiol, but which increases the incidence of uterine cancer. Dr. Lemon found that estriol, a natural, safe hormone could be used very effectively instead with far fewer side effects, and it is available in pill form.

Phyto-estrogens (plant-derived estrogen) are present in soy products. (See page 50 for the list of other sources of phyto-estrogens.) Since plant estrogens (estriol) are weak estrogens, they block the effects of excess estrogen (estrone and estradiol) in the breasts and uterus, ultimately providing protection. Plus vitamin E supplements help women's bodies make estriol.

Estrogen is not a magic pill. For some women, it could be *part* of their process through menopause. For most, a healthy diet including regular exercise is often all that a woman needs ... not for the "fountain of youth" (as claimed by the drug companies making synthetic estrogens) ... but to feel great as aging occurs, having a full life for all of your life. ▣

We are taught you must blame…It's never your fault. But it's *always* your fault, because if you wanted to change, you're the one who has got to change. It's as simple as that, isn't it?

Katheryn Hepburn

CHAPTER FOUR:
The Wrong Hormone

This chapter is based on my investigation into menopause and my resulting conclusions. This is a controversial area and your doctor may disagree with my findings. You might be tempted to automatically take your MD's word for it. Resist the temptation and read Drs. John Lee, Christiane Northrupe, and Susan Love for more detailed information. Whatever you decide to do, make the effort to be informed.

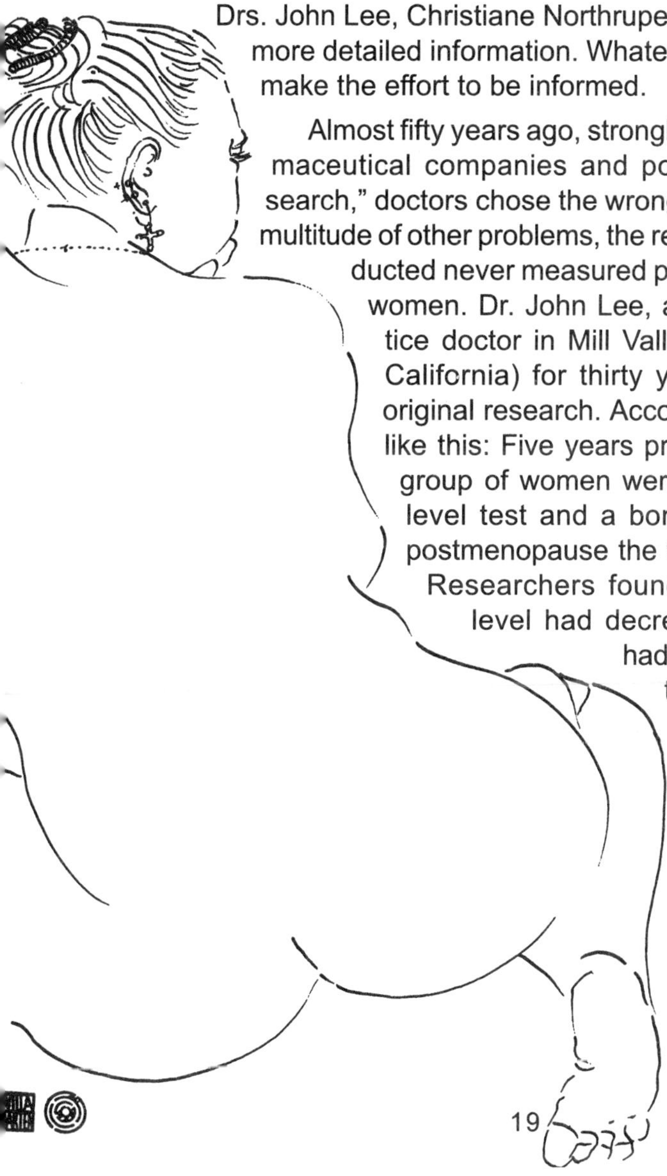

Almost fifty years ago, strongly influenced by pharmaceutical companies and poorly conducted "research," doctors chose the wrong hormone. Among a multitude of other problems, the research that was conducted never measured progesterone levels in women. Dr. John Lee, a retired family practice doctor in Mill Valley (northern coastal California) for thirty years, examined the original research. According to Lee, it looks like this: Five years prior to menopause, a group of women were given an estrogen level test and a bone scan. Five years postmenopause the tests were repeated. Researchers found that the estrogen level had decreased, osteoporosis had increased; therefore, they concluded that estrogen was the link to osteoporosis. It sounds like a logical conclusion, but they never measured the progesterone level. According to a growing number of experts, they chose the wrong hormone.

For ten years, John Lee, MD, claims to have cured osteoporosis using natural progesterone derived from wild yam. Bone is living tissue in a state of constant "remodeling." Osteoclasts are the cells that dissolve old bone, leaving a little space, which allows osteoblasts to build new bone. Some bone recycles every seven years while other bone (heel, hip) recycles every two years. If this process of breaking down and rebuilding does not occur, bone becomes brittle. It is a fragile balance. At menopause, due to diminishing progesterone, osteoblasts do not keep up with new bone development; therefore, spaces are left where new bone should be. After menopause an interference causes loss of bone mass of about 1.5% per year. Medical experts are not sure how the interference occurs. African Americans and Hispanics seem to develop osteoporosis less frequently than northern European white women do. (See Dr. Lee's book for more information.)

Underweight, smoking, drinking soda, excessive amounts of protein (more than 32–64 grams of actual protein), and not exercising all contribute to the risk of osteoporosis. It is common to see women with 30% bone loss at menopause, 50% loss at age sixty-five and a hip fracture at age 70/75 due to a missed step, not a fall. The fracture often causes the loss of independent living. Twenty-five percent of women in nursing homes with hip fractures die within two years of admittance. (A side note: The cost of hip fractures in the US is about $10 billion per year.)

Due to the original research, doctors believed that estrogen alone protected the bones and heart. It was standard procedure to prescribe estrogen therapy for menopausal women. However, in 1977, the Mayo Clinic released a warning that no one should take estrogen alone because it is an unbalanced hormone potentially causing breast and/or uterine cancer, among other things. They recommended taking it with progesterone. But if you check the PDR (Physician's Desk Reference) a full page of contra-indications, side effects, and precautions, from a loss of libido and liver cancer to acne accompanies all synthetic progesterone.

For his Ph.D. thesis, Ray Peat, a biochemist, studied the physiological effects of the hormone progesterone. He discovered that by about age forty-five, women are not ovulating. They are having periods, but their body doesn't have any more eggs, so there are none to be fertilized. Therefore, the body is no longer producing progesterone to strengthen the lining of the uterus. Women are in estrogen dominance. Age forty-five is also the time when osteoporosis accelerates. According to Dr. Peat, Dr. Lee, and many others, it is not a lack of estrogen, but a lack of progesterone that accelerates osteoporosis. Progesterone is vital to body maintenance, necessary for brain functioning, for glucose metabolism, for the thyroid hormone to be used effectively and it spurs the osteoblasts.

Further reinforcing Dr. Peat's findings, Dr. Jerrilyn Pryor, the Chief of Endocrinology in Vancouver, B.C., found that women athletes who undergo strenuous training, experience one of two phenomena: either they have periods and do not ovulate or they lose their cycle altogether. All of the women in the study had developed osteoporosis. Dr. Pryor measured both estrogen and progesterone levels. When ovulation stopped, the progesterone level dropped and osteoporosis began, even though estrogen was still being produced. She found that it is a *lack of progesterone*, not the lack of estrogen causing osteoporosis.

With all of the women taking estrogen supplements, no one has reversed osteoporosis. They have only stalled it, a bit. If estrogen were the functional hormone, we would see a reversal of osteoporosis. In addition, Tamoxifen is a drug used to block the effects of estrogen throughout the body. With ten years of use, none of the women using this drug have developed osteoporosis.

Summary

While many doctors are responsive to new information, many are reluctant to abandon a drug they have prescribed with confidence for years. They tend to resist change despite the overwhelming indications that traditional hormone replacement therapy (HRT) not only does *not* do what it claims, but also places women at greater risk for uterine and/or breast cancer. The fact is that most doctors prescribe the latest drug from research conducted by drug companies.

For more details about these and other studies, read Dr. Lee, Dr. Love, or my article in *Coast Magazine*.

... The things you refuse to meet today always come back at you later on, usually under circumstances which make the decision twice as difficult as it originally was.

Eleanor Roosevelt

CHAPTER FIVE:
What Can I Expect?

Beginning at birth, and continuing until perimenopause, the female body experiences a slow depletion of eggs. The ovaries gradually produce less estrogen and other hormones. Eventually the body runs out of eggs. As the hormone levels diminish, menstrual periods become irregular, ultimately disappearing, bones can become brittle, the risk of heart disease increases, and the vagina loses moisture and elasticity. This is all part of the aging process.

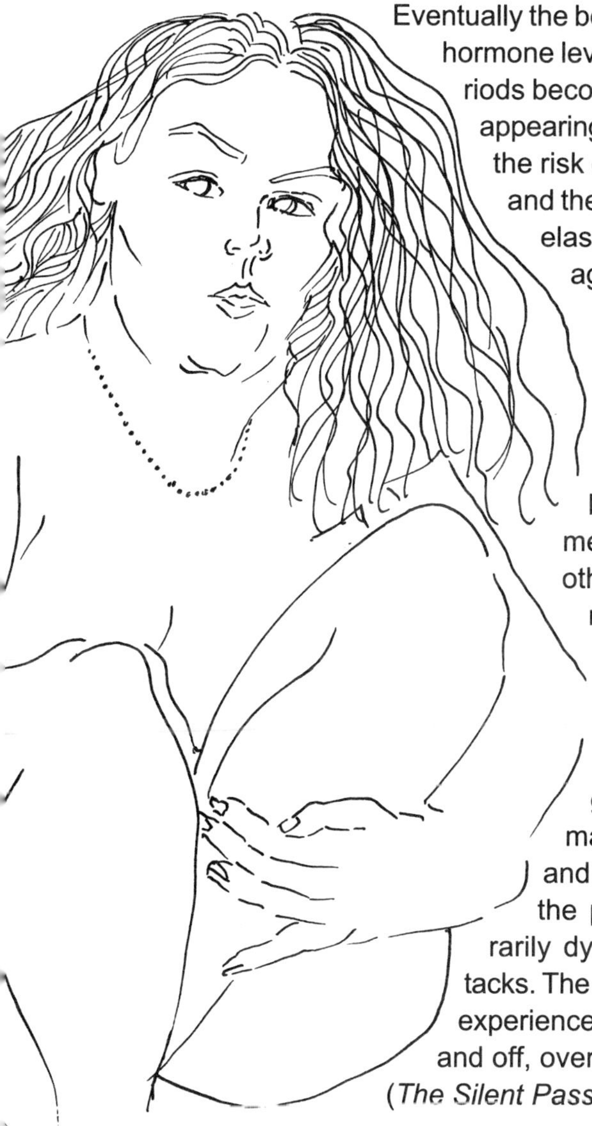

How women feel during menopause varies from woman to woman. According to many sources, about 10–15% will have little or no experience of menopausal symptoms. Another 10–15% will experience most of the symptoms of menopause: hot flashes, dramatic mood swings, night sweats, foggy thinking, vaginal dryness, migraine-like headaches, dramatic shifts between energy and fatigue, mild depression to the point of becoming temporarily dysfunctional, and panic attacks. The largest group (70–80%) will experience some of the symptoms, on and off, over a period of several years. (*The Silent Passage*)

Menopausal women who are a *little* overweight have fewer hot flashes, less vaginal dryness, and less brittle bones. There is a use for *some* fat!

Hot Flashes

Different women experience different kinds of hot flashes. Some women (at one end of the spectrum) experience a little warmth that lasts briefly and is gone as quickly as it arrives. At the other end of the spectrum, women experience profuse amounts of heat, sweat, and resulting sleep deprivation as they toss covers off, become chilled, pull them back on, only to have another hot flash and throw them back off.

Most women experience something in the middle of those two extremes: their body heats up, they flush, feel warm, and perhaps sweat; it lasts a few minutes, then passes. The worst part about hot flashes is our fear that they will happen and the fear that "people can tell." My friends and I jokingly ask, "Is it hot in here or am I having a power surge?" Even our men friends and partners joke about their own heat waves, "Can men have hot flashes? I think I'm having one right now!" Having a sense of humor about them helps you to relax and can reduce the severity and intensity of hot flashes.

Feelings

Remember puberty? I know, it was a long time ago, but sure you remember! One minute you would be calm and happy, and the next minute bouncing off the walls or crying that the world wasn't fair and nobody loved you. That is the result of an imbalance in hormones, excessive amounts of estrogen. It's true that some people experience the emotional rollercoaster throughout their lives—that may be a result of hormonal imbalance or it may be something else. Feelings of anger, bordering on rage, deep sadness and loss, and feeling in a "fog" or "cloud" are not unusual during menopause. In fact, those feelings can be quite normal. The level of rage you experience may startle you. There's nothing wrong with you for having those feelings and you may need some help surviving them (and helping those around you survive them).

Depression and panic attacks can occur as well. Women who have had hysterectomies are more likely to experience menopausal depression due to the sudden and dramatic depletion of hormones.

With regard to panic attacks, I have first hand experience and it scared me. I really thought I was going to die. I couldn't breathe and I couldn't think clearly. I felt helpless and didn't know what to do. To try to catch my breath, I ran outside, my hand on my chest, gasping for air. It was an automatic response and it happened to be the right one. The fresh, cool air calmed me and after about ten minutes, it was as if nothing had ever happened. Having treated panic attacks as a therapist, I later realized what it was. Recognizing it, understanding and knowing what to do for it makes it less frightening and more manageable.

Vaginal Dryness

Reduced estrogen levels, lack of use, and aging cause the tissue in the vagina to become thin, almost transparent, and to become dry. Despite the common misconception that women lack

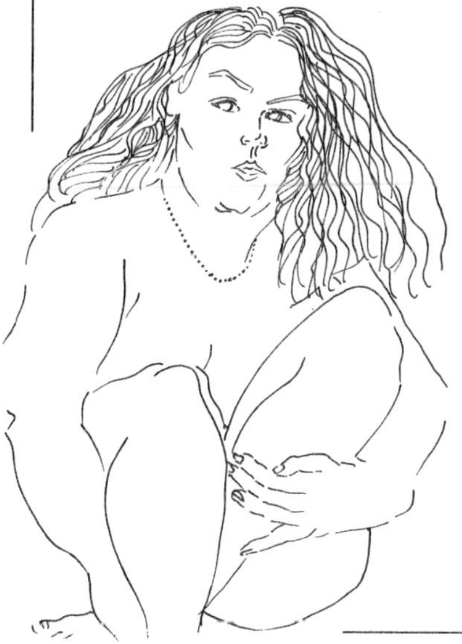

> I am learning that if I just go on accepting the framework for life that others have given me, if I fail to make my own choices, the reason for my life will be missing. I will be unable to recognize that which I have the power to change. I refuse to spend my life regretting the things I failed to do.
>
> *Liv Ullman*

interest in sex, according to women, quite the contrary seems to be true. However, one of the problems seems to be physical rather than mental or emotional. Sexual intercourse when the vagina is dry is very painful and disconcerting to both the woman and her male partner. The pain can occur throughout intercourse or just at the point that the penis is entering the vagina.

Some women do notice a change in their sex drive. Many women have experienced this as a temporary phenomenon. "Most women after the menopause ... do not experience a diminution in sex drive," according to Dr. Ramey, the senior psychologist at Georgetown University. "But a very large number do — maybe 30%," she estimates, adding that the figures are unreliable because doctors don't ask women about their sex drive. (*The Silent Passage*)

What we know is that sex drive varies from woman to woman. We also know that the drive may be there, but due to pain during intercourse women and their partners are fearful and may refrain from having sex. Other women find that their sex drive increases because they no longer worry about pregnancy.

Other Symptoms

We've discussed some of the more common symptoms of menopause; there are many others. Our bodies are getting older, our hormones are shifting, out of one balance and into another. It all takes time. Some of the other symptoms that may occur are: fluid retention, headaches, migraines, weight gain, incontinence, heavy bleeding, fibroids, dryness of the eyes and mouth, developing allergies, and constipation.

Summary

Since western culture has such a strong emphasis on female youth and beauty, menopause is linked with loss, decline, and death. There are other cultures that view the postmenopausal female as a wise woman, leader, and teacher, increasing her status, freedom, and power. In these cultures, symptoms of menopause are virtually nonexistent. (For more information read *The Silent Passage* and *Menopause, Naturally*)

Menopause is a time of change. As Susan Love explains in her hormone book, menopause is a change from our "old self" to our "new self," and "... often the anticipation of menopause is far worse than its reality," referring to a study in which 70–80% of women were relieved to reach menopause. I am one of those women, as are many of my friends.

You can expect to feel differently, to view the world through different eyes, and to experience life in an entirely new way. It is a time of loss of a role as mother; sometimes it's a loss of the role as wife; there is the loss of the ability to procreate and your body just isn't able to do what it used to do. Despite those losses, menopause can be a gift to women, a chance to re-evaluate one's life while there is time to make changes. ▣

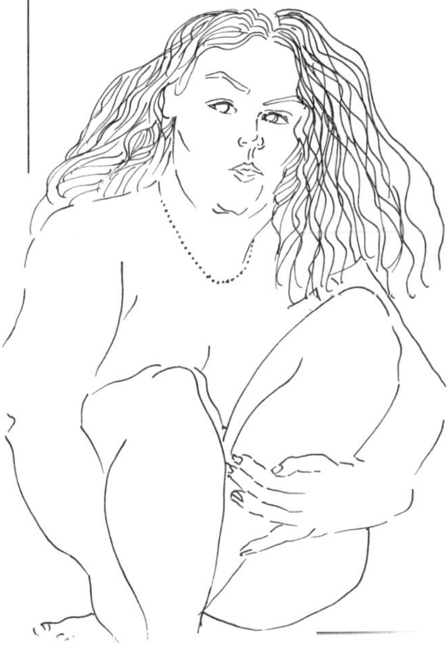

There is absolutely no point in sitting around and feeling sorry for yourself. The great power you have is to let it go ...You focus on what you have, not that which has been mean, or unkindly removed.

Minnie Driver

Throughout my life I have tried to remain true to myself. This I will continue to do as long as I live.

Jacqueline Kennedy Onassis

CHAPTER SIX:
What Is HRT?

HRT is Hormone Replacement Therapy. It means just what the words say. Usually the hormones replaced are estrogen and progesterone, and sometimes, testosterone. Your doctor, orders a blood test to check your FSH, follicle-stimulating hormone, and LH, your luteinizing hormone. (See the glossary for the definition of terms. For more in-depth information, read Drs. Love and Northrop.) As a result of these tests, your doctor prescribes hormones. You take your prescription, hoping everything will be fine now. For some it is, for others, it isn't.

The problem with measuring only the levels of FSH and LH is that they fluctuate dramatically during perimenopause. In addition to testing FSH and LH, estrogen (E), progesterone (P), and testosterone (T), DHEA, cortisol, and pregnenolone should be tested as well. Blood tests are not as reliable as saliva and urine tests for collecting this information. (See referral section in Chapter Ten for where to obtain these tests.) Many women have told me that their doctor refuses to order the tests. In that case, consider finding a doctor who wants to work *with* you. Being told that you are wrong or that you don't know what you're talking about is not helpful and doesn't facilitate increasing your knowledge about your own body.

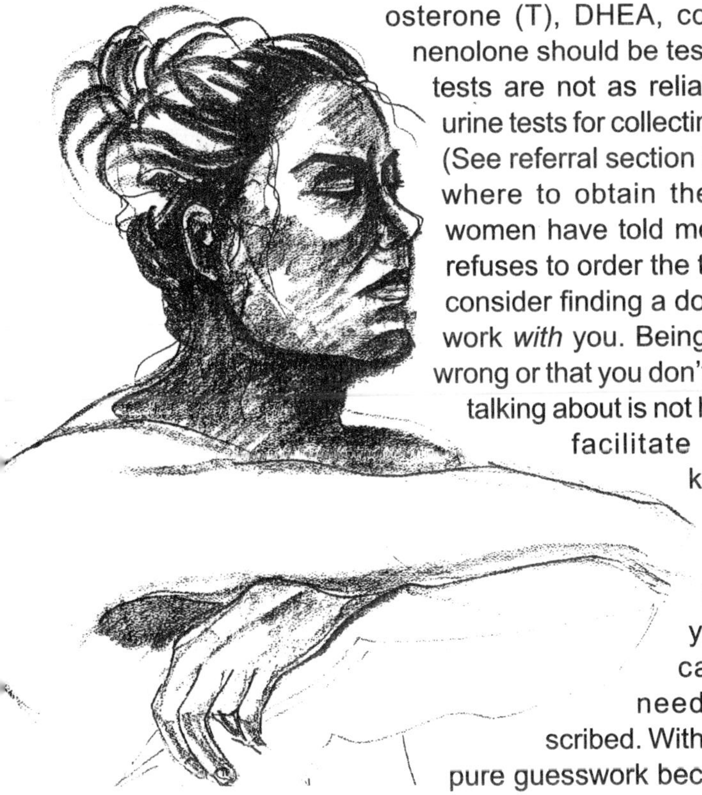

Once you have these test results, you and your doctor can decide if you need hormones prescribed. Without these tests, it's pure guesswork because each person is different. What works for one woman may not work for another. It's a good idea to have these tests taken periodically because hormones fluctuate. What works at one time, may not work at another.

The intent of replacing estrogen and other hormones is to reduce or eliminate the symptoms of menopause, to decrease the risk of heart disease, and to fend off osteoporosis. Medical experts believe that the *naturally occurring* female hormones are part of the reason why premenopausal women are far less susceptible to heart disease than men. Studies report that postmenopause, heart disease is one of the silent killers of women over fifty, responsible for over 50% of deaths among women. Osteoporosis (porous bones) is another silent killer of postmenopausal women. Whether or not HRT is "successful" in fending off these diseases is still under research since studies on hormone replacement therapy are incomplete.

One confusing issue for me, and many other women, is, if our bodies are naturally producing less estrogen, why feed it more estrogen? Because you *can* is one of the answers. The estrogen a woman's body makes keeps bones and heart healthy and strong. There is the key: *The estrogen a woman's body makes.* This estrogen is different from the chemically produced estrogen most doctors prescribe.

In 1966, gynecologist Robert Wilson's book *Feminine Forever* was published. In it he referred to menopause as "a horror ... of living decay." One-hundred-thousand books were sold within the first seven months. The book was widely excerpted in such popular women's magazines as *Vogue*. Journalists picked up on the theme so that over the late 60s and early 70s more than three hundred articles promoting estrogen replacement therapy appeared in women's magazines.

By 1975, the sale of estrogen had quadrupled; it had become one of the top five drugs sold in the US. Estrogen replacement therapy (ERT), as it was called then, was touted as the *miracle cure* for women: take it or become "sad, sexless, old crones." (*Health Magazine*, January/February 1994)

Wilson's stereotype was eventually adopted almost in its entirety by the medical profession. It has survived essentially unmodified to the present day. Sandra Coney (*The Menopause Industry: How the Medical Establishment Exploits Women*) discovered a paper bearing a title remarkably similar to that of Dr. Wilson's but published a quarter of a century later. This time it was *The Fate of the Untreated Menopause*, written by Dr. Wulf Utian and published in 1987.

In the mid-seventies, modern science realized that women on estrogen alone had eight times the risk of uterine cancer and increased risk of breast cancer. They believed that adding progesterone would reduce this risk, so they added synthetic progestin to the treatment.

Now referred to as Hormone Replacement Therapy (HRT), estrogen, progesterone, and other hormones can be replaced through the use of pills, skin patches or vaginal cream. Treatment plans for taking the combination of drugs vary; sometimes small doses of testosterone, a male hormone, are prescribed to help alleviate symptoms. The average period of time women are on HRT is about nine months mainly because the woman takes herself off of the treatment. Deciding to use HRT does not have to be permanent, a woman can change her mind at any time.

"Women wanted ERT (estrogen replacement therapy) because they were told they would age more slowly, look more attractive, and avoid the discomforts of menopause," according to Sadja Greenwood, MD, and she says doctors were looking for a quick answer to the problems of menopause. She continues, "Helping a patient clarify such problems (hot flashes, vaginal soreness, mid-life crises) takes much more time than the average doctor can spare, so prescriptions are often written as an alternative."

Surgically menopausal women (those who have had their uterus and/or ovaries surgically removed) experience a dramatic impact on their body. Instead of the gradual loss of hormones, there is a sudden and acute depletion of hormones. The need for hormone replacement therapy may be necessary to allow a gradual reduction of hormones easing the body into menopause. The question to ask your doctor is: "Do I have to use synthetic hormones or can plant-based hormones be used instead?" Perhaps use a patch instead of a pill. This would require a lower dose of estrogen and it wouldn't have to be digested thus passing through the liver. Many of the synthetic and so-called "natural" hormones like Premarin® have devastating effects on the liver.

What is happening in the United States is that women are being given HRT, increasing their estrogen dominance, which tends to increase fibroids in the uterus leading your doctor to recommend hysterectomy. In the US, one in three women have had their uterus removed. (*The Silent Passage*) Hysterectomy is the most frequently performed operation on women in the US, more than five times the number performed in Europe.

Medical doctors, who've studied the human body for years, have little more understanding about menopause than the well-informed layperson. Unfortunately since drug companies have a tremendous influence on medical training, doctors learned that menopause is a "disease" to be treated with one of the many drugs now available. At the slightest provocation, doctors dispense estrogen, as if women need to be "cured" of some disease. *Perimenopausal and menopausal women are given drugs that trick their body into thinking that they are premenopausal.*

At one time women were told that their symptoms were all in their head. Now the common belief is that *all* women will have *all* symptoms to the *same* degree and must *all* be treated with the *same* drug. Menopause has become big business.

There continues to be disagreement among the experts about the benefits and detriments of HRT. While some celebrate incomplete studies, others express caution as they expect adding progestin to the treatment will be significantly worse for the heart. The completed studies on heart disease only followed women who were taking estrogen, not combined estrogen and progestin. Many believe that progestin may counteract what they believe to be synthetic estrogen's benefits.

Some experts are optimistic. Malcolm Pike, epidemiologist at the University of Southern California, sees the benefit. He says that it really comes down to pitting one risk against another. He argues that for each breast cancer death that hormones cause, eight deaths from heart disease can be prevented. While William Castelli, director of the Farmingham Heart Project (a long-term study of cardiovascular disease) states, "This is my guess. I'll predict that progestin does not lessen the cardiovascular benefits of the estrogen in hormone therapy. But do we have that data in our hot little hands? No." (*Health Magazine*, January/February 1994) Sometimes it feels like Russian roulette using women's bodies as the target.

Two things don't make sense about all of this. First is the fact that HRT is routinely prescribed and no study has been completed on the long-term carcinogenic effects. Secondly, doctors are prescribing HRT without testing the levels of hormones already in a woman's body. Another point made by Gale Sheehy is that no progestins have been approved for hormone replacement therapy.

There are some key points that all of the experts seem to agree on. It is generally accepted that up to five years of synthetic menopausal estrogen, *probably* poses no increased risk of uterine or breast cancer. After fifteen years, your risk increases by 30%. Estrogen replacement (ERT) *claims* to reduce the risk of osteoporosis, reduce vaginal soreness and hot flashes, incontinence and mood swings. There is no documentation for those claims. There *can* be serious side effects including, but not limited to: nausea; pain, cramps, tenderness of the abdomen, breast tenderness or enlargement, blotchy skin, headaches, dizziness, changes in vision and a risk of cancer, gallbladder disease, and excessive amounts of calcium in the blood. There is *not* agreement that HRT (estrogen combined with other hormones) reduces heart disease.

Now What?

Should I take HRT or not? Good question. The answer is, "It depends." How are you feeling? If your answer is somewhere between "pretty good" and "I'm experiencing some discomforts," then read Chapter 7 and use the suggestions there as a guide through those discomforts. If you are feeling pretty uncomfortable and the suggestions in Chapter 7 don't help, then visit your health care professional. Take the saliva test. (That's its "technical" name!) When you receive the results, ask for a copy and keep them in a file. Believe it or not, you will want to refer to them.

If your doctor is talking about HRT before ever seeing test results, you need a new doctor, *now*. When you schedule your doctor's appointment, be sure to let them know that you will need more time with the doctor. Don't accept a booklet (especially one created by a drug company) instead of *time to talk with your doctor!* Ask your doctor about menopause, what it is, how they view it, the best approach to it, their attitude about the process, what they think your attitude should be, and discuss societal attitudes that influence individual attitudes. Talk about it so you know that you are speaking the same language. If your doctor doesn't spend time talking to you about this, you need a different doctor. I know they are busy people, so are you. You are important and you deserve the time and the support through this important transition. You are paying them for their time!

Ask your doctor about natural (plant-derived) hormones, rather than synthetic hormones, like Premarin®, the most "popular" brand. (For more information, see the next section in this chapter: About the So-Called "Natural" Hormones.) Start with natural hormones that are not chemically processed. If those don't work, then try the ones that are plant-derived, natural hormones that have been chemically processed. There is rarely a reason to use synthetic hormones. I say rarely because experts whom I trust have told me that there are occasions when synthetic hormones are necessary for a "short" time, a maximum of five years. Remember that HRT is the exception, not the rule!

About the So-Called "Natural" Hormones

Premarin® is the tradename for the most "popular" pill used in HRT. The estrogen is extracted from pregnant mares. The name Premarin® means pregnant mare urine, PMU. According to a 1994 report in *Equus Magazine*: "From October through March—the period of highest estrogen production—each mare is hooked up around the clock to a harness attached to a funnel that collects the urine and carries it down a tube into a one gallon container. Urine sells for $12 to $17 per gallon." Consequently cash-strapped farmers are clamoring for a piece of the action. More than one thousand potential PMU farmers are on a waiting list. There has been a great deal of discussion and debate about the treatment of the horses. They are hooked up to a catheter-like device in stalls so small, they cannot move. The results are severe leg problems from endless hours of standing. Since these animals are only bred for their urine, the results are that annually, somewhere between forty and sixty-five thousand foals are sold for slaughter.

Initially, the government regulated the conditions on the farms, but that has changed. According to Ayerst, the manufacturer of Premarin® , we should be assured that things have improved, the animals are being treated more humanely now that Ayerst, instead of the government, is responsible for overseeing the humane treatment of the horses. Personally, I do not find comfort in this notion.

PETA, People for Ethical Treatment of Animals, is calling for a boycott of products made by Ayerst and their parent company, American Products Corp. The products include: Chef Boyardee, Advil, Dristan, and Jiffy Pop.

Summary

If you decide to use HRT, try a patch or cream. When taking a pill, you have to take a higher dose because so much of the benefit is lost as the pill passes through your system. In addition, experts agree that HRT in the pill form is much harder on the liver.

If you decide to use HRT, it does not have to be a permanent decision. *You can change your mind.* Seriously consider the effects of long term use of synthetic hormones.

Remember that the purpose of HRT is to *help* our bodies with the transition from child-bearing to non-child-bearing, from monthly periods to no periods, from higher doses of naturally-occurring hormones to lower levels; *helping* our bodies *ease* into the natural next step, menopause.

All of the experts, despite their strong beliefs pro or con HRT, agree that women need to ask questions, understand the implications of HRT, and decide the best approach, based on family history, information gathered by reading and talking with their doctor and other women, and their own personal preferences. There is no question that popping a pill is easier. The real question is: Is it better for your health and well being both short and long term? Only you can answer that question. ▣

Redefine the word "fail." There is no failure in life other than not trying. If you want something badly enough, make an attempt. If you want to paint, get a brush and do it. If you want to sing, sing. A lot of people get scared. They're afraid to fail. Take that word out of your vocabulary. You didn't "fail." You "tried your best."

Jane Seymour

CHAPTER SEVEN:
Alternatives to HRT

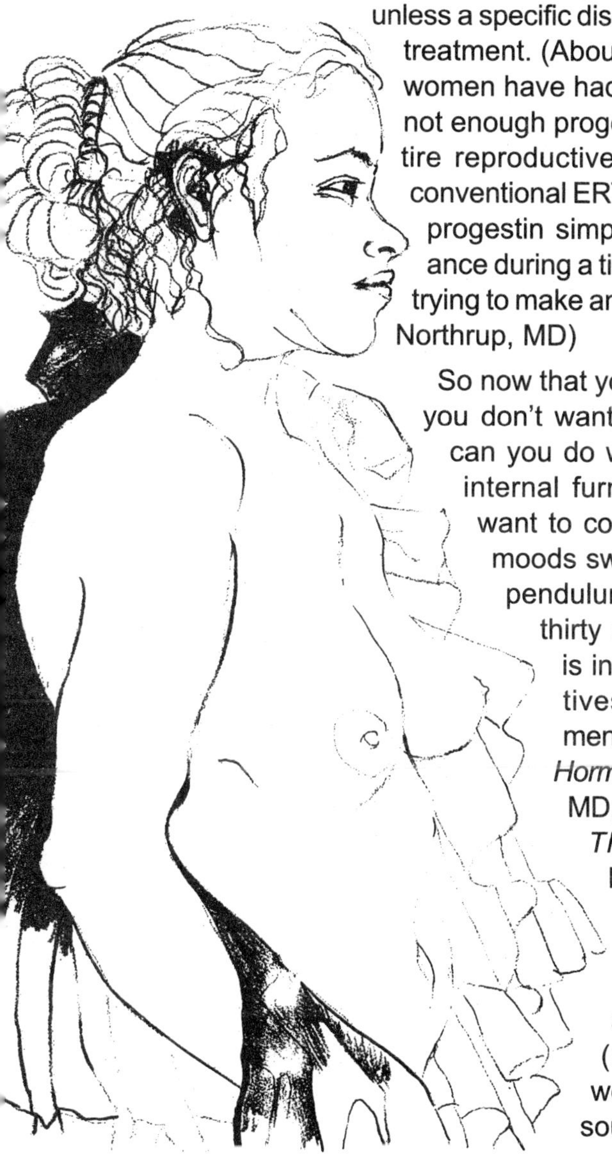

In 1981, the World Health Organization came to the conclusion that menopause is a natural part of aging and requires no treatment unless a specific disease or symptom needed treatment. (About time!) "Many American women have had too much estrogen and not enough progesterone during their entire reproductive lives. Putting them on conventional ERT regimens with synthetic progestin simply re-creates this imbalance during a time when their bodies are trying to make an adjustment." (Christiane Northrup, MD)

So now that you think maybe, perhaps you don't want to use HRT/ERT, what can you do when, for example, your internal furnace heats up and you want to cool down? Or when your moods swing from one end of the pendulum to the other in about thirty seconds? The following is information about alternatives to HRT and ERT for menopausal symptoms. *The Hormone Book* by Susan Love, MD; *The Menopausal Years, The Wise Woman Way* by Susun S. Weed; Dr. Gary Klepper, Dr. Lois Johnson, Joanna Baird Mallouk, Dr. John Lee, and personal experience (mine and many other women's) are the primary sources of this information.

Wild Yam

In the 40s, wild yam was found to reduce menopausal symptoms, in particular hot flashes, but the pharmaceutical companies could not find a way to patent it, so they turned to synthetic, patentable hormones (Dr. John Lee, *What Your Doctor Won't Tell You About Menopause*). Fifty years later, however, wild yam has become one of the more popular approaches to reducing the discomforts of menopause. Now it seems that everybody is making some form of wild yam cream. Drs. Lee and Love in their respective books have a list of what they consider high quality yam cream. I've added MoonMaid Botanicals Pro-Meno to their list.

Dr. Lee claims to have cured osteoporosis by having his patients use natural progesterone from wild yam. Patients were given bone density tests pre-treatment and again during treatment to measure the changes in density. Using a program that included natural progesterone cream, diet, mineral and vitamin supplements, and modest exercise, Dr. Lee was able to reverse osteoporosis in all of his patients who were following this regime.

Not all wild yam creams are created equal! Some wild yam is chemically processed into progesterone cream, while other products are simply the wild yam in varying concentrations. Pro-Gest is one of the more popular brands of chemically treated creams. Many women are very pleased with the results of using Pro-Gest. Others have had serious skin eruptions (which was my experience) and others developed an excess of progesterone in their systems. Pro-Gest now makes wild yam oil that they claim does not cause skin eruptions.

MoonMaid Botanicals makes a wild yam cream called Pro-Meno which contains wild yam plus vitex, black cohosh, and licorice root, necessary for women who are getting too many estrogens from other sources (in particular meat and dairy products). Personally, I use MoonMaid; they use high quality oils, flower essences, grapefruit seed extract with vitamin E as a preservative. When I read their label, I know exactly what I am getting and I have met the woman who creates the product. (See Chapter 9 for their number.) Anecdotally, women report great success using Pro-Meno from elimination of hot flashes and mood swings to reduction or elimination of fibroids in their uterus. Find the wild yam cream that's right for you.

The medical community would argue with me that our bodies could not make progesterone from wild yam cream. They claim to know this because they have tested it. What I do know is that I haven't ovulated in seven years (which means my body makes little or no progesterone). After using Pro-Meno for several years, I took the four-day saliva test from Great Smokies Laboratories and I have tons of progesterone. (My four-day range — over a two-week period of time — was between 150 and 427 — average is 53 to 193. The test involves spitting into a tube on the first, fifth, ninth, and thirteenth days and sending each tube into Great Smokies Lab for testing.) As a result of this test, my doctor asked me to stop using the Pro-Meno. She found it hard to believe that my progesterone was that high due to the Pro-Meno cream, but, as she says, nothing would surprise her any more! I stopped using the cream for a full month, then I was re-tested. The results were a dramatic drop in my progesterone level, a range of 105 to 221. To really test it, I should have stayed off of it longer.

As I mentioned in Chapter 4, the medical community chose the wrong hormone for treatment of menopausal symptoms. This error continues today. Medical doctors automatically prescribe estrogen for their patients instead of testing their hormones to find out what they actually need.

Horsetail, Anyone?

If you live in a moist climate, you have probably found an overabundance of horsetail (equisetum) in your garden. Spring is the perfect time to pick horsetail. Its healing qualities seem to be extensive. Joanna Baird Mallouk explains that horsetail is 70% water-soluble silica, which is also found in all the cells of the body. It finds its way to the bone and strengthens it. It also makes nails strong (soak your nails in it) and hair glossy (use it as a rinse). Both Joanna and Susun Weed recommend it for hot flashes. And all three sources (plus several others) agree that horsetail tea made from fresh or dried spring-gathered horsetail is excellent to heal and strengthen bone in the human body. It is said to help reverse osteoporosis.

To make the tea, place the rinsed horsetail in a jar and pour boiling water over it. The ratio is one ounce of horsetail to eight ounces (a cup) of boiled water. Allow it to steep for 15–20 minutes. You can make large amounts at one time and store the left over beverage in the refrigerator. For hot flashes drink one cup, three times a day for a week, then don't drink it the next week. Continue alternating weeks until the hot flashes stop. For osteoporosis, drink one glass a day.

There are problems with horsetail. One potential side effect from horsetail is if you are borderline in B1 reserves, this herb could create a deficiency. Consequently, you would be wise to supplement with a complex B containing B1. Warning: *If you experience sensations of nervous sensitivity or urinary irritability after drinking it, don't use it.* It is always best to talk to your health care professional before taking herbs with potential side effects.

Power Surges

So far, two remedies for power surges (hot flashes) have been suggested: horsetail and wild yam cream. There is a third option which many women have found helpful. GLA, gamma linolenic acid, obtained from evening primrose, borage, and black currant oil can be extremely beneficial in alleviating or minimizing hot flashes. All three (horsetail, wild yam, and GLA) are available through your health food store and many pharmacies now carry a large selection of supplements. I found taking three or four softgels of 135 mg of GLA per day made a dramatic difference in my hot flashes. You may need to experiment with increasing the GLA, wild yam cream, and vitamins E and C to alleviate your hot flashes and fuzzy thinking.(See chart on page 50 for good sources of vitamins E and C.)

Many of the pharmaceutical companies are coming out with new products (almost by the minute, or so it seems). Many of these products have the word menopause in the name. As with HRT, not all doses are correct for all women. We are not all alike! Talk with your health care professional, s/he can work with you to find out what is missing in your diet and help you design a supplement program that works for you!

Incontinence

A common problem for menopausal women is the weakening of the pelvic floor muscles. According to Jeannette Brown, MD, in the *San Francisco Focus*, September 1994, incontinence is a "don't ask, don't tell" problem—women don't tell their doctors and doctors don't ask.

For stress incontinence (losing urine when you laugh, cough, sneeze), Kegel exercises are still the best "medicine." (Exercise is good for you, period.) There are studies that have shown these exercises help strengthen the PC (pubococcygeal) muscle. The PC muscle is the one you use to control your urine. You can find it by simply stopping yourself from urinating. *That* is the muscle you need to exercise. Do short quick squeezes of one second on, one second off; then longer squeezes of three seconds on, three seconds off; then squeeze for ten seconds, rest for ten. The experts suggest doing about two hundred per day. The beauty of them is that you can do them anywhere and no one knows that you are exercising. You can easily make them part of your routine.

For frequency and urgency problems, see your health care professional. Kegel exercises may help with them and there may be a physical problem that needs to be addressed.

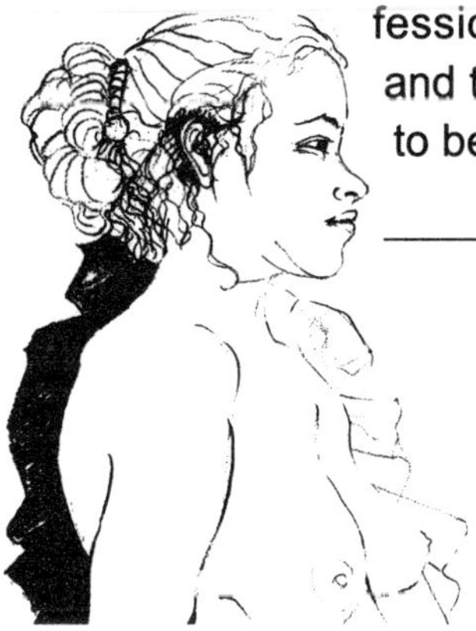

See into life – don't just look at it.

Anne Baxter

Feelings, Thoughts, and Emotions

If your thinking is fuzzy, there are a number of alternative approaches that have been studied and recommended. The obvious ones are decrease smoking, alcohol, and caffeine use, eat a balanced diet, and exercise. There are two basic kinds of exercise. Physical exercise increases reaction time and blood flow to the brain. Exercise the brain by going back to school, learn a new language, join a book club, and challenge your mind. The premise is "use it or lose it." With regard to herbs, Susun Weed's book and Michael Murray's *The Healing Power of Herbs*, discuss sage, ginseng, and ginkgo bilboa to help sharpen thinking.

As I mentioned in Chapter 5, panic attacks could be a symptom of menopause. The most important thing to remember is that it will go away. This is not a permanent life situation. A little knowledge about panic attacks can help minimize or alleviate them. Talk to your friends or partner about these feelings so they can help you through them. Isolating yourself will only make matters worse. Personally, if panicky feelings begin to rise in my chest now, I take deep breaths and go outside. Drinking water also helps, lots of water. Now I can say, "Oh, so that's part of menopause for me, hmmm? OK. I can handle it."

Occasionally, I experience a feeling of restlessness and discomfort: I may be at my computer writing, or gardening or eating a meal. I automatically think that I have to do something *now*. My tendency has been to take a walk, drink water, the usual. It happened not long ago while flying across country. I couldn't very well go for a walk. Fortunately, I was in the middle of reading Rebecca Latimer's book and I remembered what she said about meditating. So I began to meditate immediately. I don't know how long it took since I didn't time myself, but it couldn't have been very long, maybe ten minutes, and I felt back to "normal." So I've added meditation to my list of to-dos. I'm trying to meditate as a way of feeling calm and grounded plus alleviating those restless, uncomfortable feelings before they start.

I don't want to minimize the feelings that can surface during this time. Knowing that it is temporary can really help. Having a group of women friends (or a women's support group) can help too. Our western cultural attitudes about menopause, exercise, diet (as in the food we eat, not dieting) are wreaking havoc on our bodies as we go through "the change." Keeping a journal helped me to find patterns and understand myself better. It doesn't have to be rigid or daily, just a notebook in which to write thoughts, feelings, reflections, words for your eyes only. Going back to read them periodically can help you realize that things are changing.

Vaginal Dryness and Loss of Elasticity

As the vagina looses moisture and elasticity, sexual intercourse with a man can be very painful. As the penis enters the vagina, the woman experiences pain that can be anything from mild to fairly severe. Many women have found that once the penis is inside, the pain subsides and sex is very enjoyable. This pain can be awful and difficult to get past. With a sensitive partner who is willing to take time, experiment, and help you, sex can be very pleasurable.

Again remember the old adage "use it or lose it"? It is very true in this case. Whether you are having sex with a partner (male or female) or masturbating, activity helps the elasticity and moisture of the vagina.

If the dryness you experience is mild, you can use one of the alternatives to synthetic estrogen creams (which can have side effects, as well as, being absorbed by your partner during intercourse). MoonMaid Botanicals all natural Vital Vulva (I love the name) can be applied to the vagina. Use it at night just before bed, your vagina will absorb it as you sleep. By the way, many women have found it to be extremely beneficial for helping the elasticity of the soft tissue around the eyes.

Women's Health Institute Lubricating Gel is free of hormones, safe to use, may be used during intercourse, and is a good moisturizer for the vagina. Or place a vitamin E softgel inside your vagina each night for six weeks, then once a week after that. Using one of these forms of lubrication (or finding another type that works for you) can be extremely beneficial to minimize or alleviate pain. Even if you find that the opening to your vagina is moist, inside may not be. Try using a lubricant. You (and your partner) may be pleasantly surprised.

If these suggestions do not work, you may need an estrogen cream. As noted in Chapter 3, not all estrogens are alike. Using creams containing estriol can be very beneficial. The low-dose cream (about .05 milligrams of estriol) is applied to the inside of the vagina (with an applicator) nightly for two weeks, then two or three times a week thereafter. There are also tinctures, teas, and dry herbs that contain phyto-estrogens and can alleviate pain during intercourse.

If none of these methods work, there are chemically processed estrogens that you can use. Talk to your health care professional about these. Remember, phyto-estrogens are plant-based estrogens, easier on your system than synthetic estrogens. Again, get tested to find out what hormones are missing. It may not be estrogen that you need.

Many women have said that they have given up on sex because it is so painful. With your partner, get creative. Until intercourse is comfortable again, there are many creative ways to have sex. Use your imagination! Have fun! Try something new! You and your partner may be pleasantly surprised! You deserve to have a good sex life.

Skin Eruptions

No where in any of the literature can I find anything about this. This information is strictly based on discussions with menopausal and postmenopausal women. In talking to women I discovered that many of them were getting itchy bumps on their elbows and/or lower back near the spine. Their experiences all seemed to be the same and nothing seemed to effect these irritations. They began as rough spots, then became bumps, turned red, began to itch, and eventually dried up, became scaly and went away, only to return again several weeks later. Calendula, comfrey, antibiotic creams or ointments, even Lotrimin didn't work. When I asked my holistic doctor about this, he suggested using a body brush (not a luffa or sponge) to scrub your entire body every time you bathe. This is the only thing that worked.

I don't know how many women this effects, but I spoke with enough women that it made me realize that I needed to mention it.

Life-Style Changes

I preface this section with a quote from Rebecca Latimer, as she urges us to add fifteen minutes of meditation per day, for our own good. She says, "It is a hard fact that if you want to make the most of your old age, you probably will have to change, and change doesn't come easily or painlessly. You will need to apply self-discipline. You may think that it's too late for you to change yourself, that your habits are too deeply rooted, that you are too old to experiment with odd and difficult exercises, but I must tell you that I don't think anyone is too old to change, just as I think anyone can learn a new skill at any age." (Latimer was ninety-one when she finished her book.)

Every expert agrees that if you smoke or drink heavily (alcohol, more than one drink per day, and caffeine, more than two cups per day), you should stop or *at least* cut back. Either can be toxic to your bone cells and reduce your body's absorption of calcium. Also, peri-, post- and menopausal women need to watch the amount of protein, especially from meat, as it increases the body's acidity. In order for the body to maintain the proper pH, it depletes calcium directly from the bones. Many women who eat meat with hormones in it find that their hot flashes and mood swings increase. Even post-menopausal women who haven't had a hot flash in years suddenly begin to have them following several days of eating meat and/or dairy with hormones.

Exercise, ideally weight bearing, at least three times a week for 20–30 minutes each time, can decrease the risk of osteoporosis. (Exercising for longer period of time provides more benefit.) Adding up to 1500 mg. of calcium plus 100–400 mg. of magnesium per day helps too. Magnesium is a critical part of the picture. Some experts claim that magnesium is more crucial than calcium. Women who begin exercise and supplements in their early 30s build strong bones as a good base prior to menopause. Women in their 40s, 50s, 60s, and so on, can markedly improve their bone structure.

Reduce or eliminate processed sugar from your diet. It seems that everything has sugar in it. I noticed that my hot flashes were far worse when I ate sugar. Eliminating processed sugar and only eating foods with small amounts of pure maple syrup or fructose were easier for me to digest and didn't cause my body heat to rise. This is a time when it is important to pay attention to how food, people, and life effect you. Try to avoid that which affects you negatively. For several years, I had to avoid all alcohol; even organic wines gave me hot flashes. Now I can drink a glass or two of wine with dinner and experience no ill effects.

Vitamin supplementation may need to be a part of your life style change. Throughout this chapter are suggestions of what to supplement and why. In addition to those, several sources recommend taking 50% more magnesium than calcium for up to three months for hormone imbalance. They indicate that this will increase your energy and reduce tension. It is a favorite supplement for naturopathic physicians in treating premenstrual syndrome.

Drink plenty of water throughout the day. If you find that you rise often during the night to relieve yourself, drink most of your water before 3 PM. Avoid stimulants, fad foods, and fad diets.

Consistently, women tell me that the message they are getting from their bodies is to slow down during perimenopause and after. Experts reinforce this notion. Take more time for yourself. Let go of some of your projects. Take time at home, alone. Pay attention to you and your body. Take walks on the beach or in the woods or even around the block. Consider taking vacation with a group of women friends. With the help of friends, loved ones, and/or a therapist find what fits for you, whether it is exercise, diet, time alone or with others. This is the beginning of the second half of your life, and it's about you.

Stronger Bones and Heart

If you want to know your bone density level, there are relatively simple and inexpensive tests available. Dual Photon bone density test (DPA) and the dual energy x-ray (DEXA) can measure bone density within 98% accuracy. Doctors make use of the test to know that their patient's treatment is working.

Calcium is a strong support for proper osteoblast/osteoclast functioning. Where does calcium come from? Naturally the first thought is dairy products (from cows). But where do cows get it? From the plants they eat. It is in the stalks, stems, and leaves. It's what gives the plants the strength to hold themselves up. If you eat the plants, nutrition experts explain, it is a much more efficient way to obtain calcium. Plus a large portion of the population is allergic to dairy products. (See list of calcium-rich foods on page 50.)

Eat a diet rich in calcium. As you get older, take supplements of calcium citrate or lactate, which are the easiest type of calcium for the body to assimilate. Calcium carbonate is the most popular because it is the cheapest to produce; it is also less beneficial and difficult for the human body to absorb.

Some experts recommend beginning to supplement with calcium capsules at about age thirty-five. Up to 1500 milligrams per day is recommended. Dr. Klepper of The Ninth Wave, cautions against taking calcium carbonate (like Tums, oyster shell, dolomite) as they can carry significant amounts of lead. He also recommends adding magnesium to balance the calcium, warning that "too much calcium alone can induce cramping." You may need other supplements to increase the absorption of calcium.(See page 50 for magnesium-rich foods.) It's a good idea to seek treatment from a specialist who knows how to test your muscles (applied kinesiology) in order to let you know exactly what *your* body requires.

In order for calcium to be absorbed, there must be sufficient hydrochloric acid (stomach acid to absorb food) and vitamin D. As people approach ages 65–70, their stomach isn't producing much hydrochloric acid. According to Dr. Klepper, if you take your age less 10, it indicates your chances of having reduced stomach acid.

For example, if you are a 60 year old, subtract 10, that leaves 50; you have a 50% chance of having reduced stomach acid and therefore needing to supplement with hydrochloric acid, HCl. You will know that your stomach is working inefficiently if you experience heartburn, bloating, burping, or a heavy feeling following a meal. If most of your meal is still in your stomach about forty-five minutes later, your stomach is probably working inefficiently. Supplements of HCl can be bought at health food stores. Capsules are less irritating than pills. Take them with a warm or hot beverage during your meal to help them dissolve more easily. Start with one pill and increase gradually up to three or four per meal.

Skin, with the sun's help, makes vitamin D, but we wear clothes. Dr. Lee suggests that 99% of women are vitamin D deficient. According to him, we need one to two hours a day nude in the sun or we can take supplements. (Given the risk of skin cancer, supplements sound like the wise woman's route, although other experts report that 45 minutes in the morning would provide the vitamin D needed.)

Some other supplements to consider follow: Boron is instrumental in calcium metabolism, aiding in the absorption of both calcium and magnesium. Copper slows the breakdown of bone and helps with bone repair. Manganese is needed for cartilage and to stimulate compounds found in the bone. Selenium is also necessary for components in the bone. Silicon helps the bone structure that supports calcification. Zinc helps create osteoblasts, osteoclasts, and bone proteins while assisting in bone repair and in vitamin D function.

An important factor in reducing the risk of osteoporosis is avoiding excessive amounts of protein, that is, more than 32–64 grams per day (depending on your weight and age). Excessive animal protein cannot be stored; consequently, it is excreted through the kidneys, causing them to lose calcium. Your body replaces lost calcium by leaching it from the bones. Sodas with phosphorus (like Coke and Pepsi) do the same thing; *the phosphorus leaches calcium from the bones.*

Coenzyme Q10 (CoQ10) is an enzyme that is made in the human body and diminishes after about the age of thirty. Heart, liver, muscle, brain, and other vital organs all require CoQ10 to produce ATP, the body's main energy storage molecule. CoQ10 is also needed by another key enzyme, which turns both carbohydrates and fat into usable energy. A powerful antioxidant, CoQ10 protects cholesterol in the blood from oxidation damage. Processed carbohydrates are not good sources of CoQ10. See the chart on page 50 for the best sources of CoQ10. Supplementing CoQ10 is probably the best way to assure that you are taking the necessary amount. The recommended dosage is 100 mg. per day of rice oil-based CoQ10 or 250 mg. of powdered.

Food is an important part of maintaining strong bones and heart. Hundreds of books and articles have been written on the subject. Make a point of reducing the number of meat meals and using organic meats in order to avoid the estrogens and antibiotics in non-organic animal products. While protein is important, too much protein can be very hard on the system. Creating a balance is the key here.

As we age, the ability of the body to digest animal products drops dramatically. If you eat animal products, eat a small amount at one sitting; chew your food completely before swallowing it. You can increase the quality of the protein you eat by making bone soup. Using bone from organic or free-range animals and cooking it in water for twenty-four hours cooks all the nutrients out of the bone and into the broth. You can freeze part of the broth and save it for future use. It becomes the base for any soup you make. Vary the kind of animal you use for the broth. Fish also makes wonderful nutritious broth. Cook the fish including the bone and remove or strain the bone prior to adding other ingredients.

Remember the main purpose of food is to nourish your body. (Though I am certainly not opposed to great tastebud treats!) In this rushed world of ours, people tend to gobble food over business lunches and dinners. Meals need to be a time to relax.

If you want more information about why we should eat organic products, read books by John Robbins, Marc Lappé or Francine Lappé. It's frightening and cause for alarm to realize what the poultry, cattle, and dairy industry are using to "feed" animals.

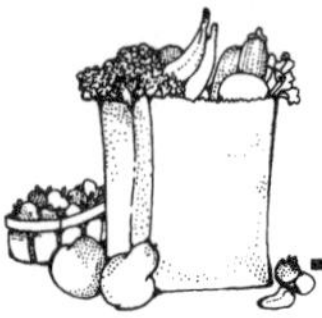

Foods That Can Help

Sources of
B COMPLEX

Asparagus
Avocado
Quinoa
Salmon
Soy food

Sources of
BIOFLAVINOIDS

Citrus fruit
Cherries
Grapes
Soy food

Sources of
VITAMIN C

Orange
Guava
Cooked spinach
Raw spinach
Cantaloupe
Mango
Grapefruit juice
Strawberry
Watermelon
Cooked cauliflower
Raw cauliflower
Cooked broccoli
Raw broccoli
Green pepper
Red pepper
Kiwi
Grapefruit
Asparagus
Orange juice

Sources of
CALCIUM

Canned fish
with edible bones
(salmon, sardines)
Carob bar
Rhubarb
Dandelion greens
Collard greens
Chinese cabbage
Kale
Cooked spinach
Tofu
Mustard greens
Tempeh
Broccoli
Mussels
Oysters
Miso
Soybeans
Lobster
Navy beans
Almonds

Sources of
CoQ10

Organ meat -
liver, kidney, heart
Muscle meats
Fish
Peanuts
Spinach
Soy
Nuts

Sources of
VITAMIN E

Asparagus
Avocado
Mango
Sunflower seeds
Wheat germ oil

Sources of
MAGNESIUM

Asparagus
Artichoke
Avocado
Bananas
Lima beans
Navy beans
Black beans
Bran
Broccoli
Haddock
Nuts
Oatmeal
Peas
Baked potatoes
Brown rice
Soybeans
Soy food
Spinach
Yogurt

Sources of
PHYTOESTROGENS

Soy food
Tofu
Soy milk
Roasted soy butter
Soy protein powder
Canned or frozen
soybeans
Fresh soybeans
(edamame)
Tempeh
Roasted soy nuts

Exercise

Here's that exercise thing again. Exercise is a critical factor for strong bones, heart, and a healthy body and mind. Experts agree that a minimum of 20–30 minutes at least three times a week of weight-bearing exercise will dramatically reduce the risk of osteoporosis. (I know I'm repeating myself, but I cannot emphasize this enough!) Weight-bearing means using at least light weights, 1–3 pounds. It's important to put stress on your body. (The good kind, not "the kids are driving me nuts" or "I had a rotten day at the office" kind.) It can also reduce cholesterol and strengthen the functioning of the heart. Make it a fun activity instead of drudgery. If jogging is not your thing, then don't do it, because you'll quit in a few weeks. I've found that varying my activity works. I love to dance, so I bit the bullet and began dancing at forty-five—jazz, tap, ballet, funk. I felt like an elephant, at first. It was painful and a struggle to stay in class. I cried many times even during class. I stayed with it because something about it felt right for me. Now I perform, am comfortable looking at my body in the mirror, and have even been told that I'm a pretty good dancer. Seven years later, I still love it!

It's been a joy to watch my body change. I swim and take yoga twice a week. I've found that activities with other people help to motivate and encourage me to maintain my exercise regime. Get a friend to make a commitment with you so you can support and encourage each other. Set accomplishable goals for yourself and reward your successes. Design a program that *works for you!* One that you will actually do! Make a list of physical activities that you enjoy. Pick one every other day or three or four times a week.

Migraines and Headaches

Even if you've never had a headache or a migraine in your life, you may start having them as your hormones struggle to rebalance. Some of the worst may occur during your periods. Here are a number of possible remedies to try. They've all been successfully used and some may work better for you than others.

Try using lavender oil, a good quality one (Jurlique and Trinity both make a very good one; Aura Cacia is pretty good). Put a drop of oil on a facial tissue and inhale it. If the migraine has taken hold, put a drop on the inside of your wrist or elbow where your veins are closer to the surface to get the oil into your blood stream more quickly. Take a drop and rub it into the base of your skull or better yet, ask your partner to do that for you. You can also purchase an inhaler, which dissipates the oil into the air you breathe. Start this treatment at the first hint of a headache. However, if lavender oil doesn't smell good to you, don't use it.

Cold compresses on the painful side of your face and neck, preferably before the pain becomes unbearable. Keep changing the compress to make sure it is cool.

Sex. Surprised? You know the cartoons where the woman says, "Not now, honey, I have a headache." Sex is a great tension reliever. Headaches are often related to stress and tension. "Honey, I have a headache," can have new meaning for you and your partner.

Cranial sacral adjustments, acupuncture, and massage are also very effective with long term success. In some cases, it may take several sessions before you notice a change. All of these are part of taking care of yourself, nurturing your body.

The next section is part of reducing headaches and migraines. Taking care of you and reducing stress will make the passage through menopause easier.

Reducing Stress

It is important to take time for yourself, especially as you enter menopause. A woman's life is devoted to caring for others. The children left home, you and your partner are nearing retirement; it's time to take time for you. What is it that you want for the second half of your life?

Joanna Baird Mallouk's attitude about menopause is, "If someone has given you a lot of hype about menopause and you believe it, then you are probably going to have trouble. As you are nearing menopause, it's an important time to back off of things, don't get into the trap of adding stressful jobs to your life. I don't suffer stress because I work it off. I'm constantly working things off. If you stress about things, you'll definitely have a harder time. So if something is causing you stress, get rid of it ... even if it's your husband. Hopefully, it isn't that drastic!"

For years I've heard people talking about meditating to relieve stress. I tried it a couple of times and felt very unsuccessful. In her book, Rebecca Latimer talks about learning to meditate as a way to relax, reduce tension, and feel more grounded. She says, "I have to admit, I'm a lousy meditator. But I can testify that even such a poor performer is changed. I myself had a friend remark on it. (My husband!)" So now I've begun to meditate ten minutes a day. I'm a poor performer too *and* I notice the difference. I feel calmer, more centered and relaxed.

The key is to take more time for you. You deserve it! Make dates with yourself, write them in your appointment book and when someone tries to schedule during your time tell them, "No, I already have a commitment that can't be changed." Once taking time for you becomes a habit, you will guard and cherish it as if it were gold.

Once a month, I meet with a small group of women whom I adore! We meet for three hours and share pieces of ourselves with each other. There is a lot of support given and received. I can't imagine not having my monthly sanctuary. We recently planned a three-day retreat at my house. My wonderful husband graciously agreed to stay away from home for those days. The other group members' partners agreed to take care of kids and household during our retreat. There was only one emergency call the entire time! We've decided to make this an annual event and perhaps even go out of town.

I've added a weekly gathering for one hour with another group of women friends. We get together at 4:30 PM at a local meeting place to take a break from our responsibilities and to talk and laugh. None of us are allowed to talk about work, our jobs, our kids, or our partners during this time. It's a wonderful treat for all of us. When I miss it, I really miss it!

It's all a part of creating a balance in our lives. It's a fragile balance between self, partner, friends, children, other family members, career, volunteer work, and all kinds of commitments. If it isn't balanced, all of those parts lose. Be good to yourself. Take time for you because you're worth it! ▣

Challenges make you discover things about yourself that you never really knew. They're what makes the instrument stretch—what makes you go beyond the norm.

Cicely Tyson

CHAPTER EIGHT:
Summary

Many of us are scared to say the "m" word, as if saying the word will cause wrinkles to appear! Our mothers were certainly never encouraged to mention it, but this isn't a cold or flu nor is it cancer. The body is simply shifting into another phase of life, *that's all.* Any shift or change *can* be painful and difficult. Anyone who's ever made any kind of a change in their life knows how tough change can be. Anyone who's been in therapy knows that even change for the good is painful. Your body is no longer what it was; it is evolving. Feel it, understand it, and learn to accept it. This is a time of powerful change, grieving and a loss of the old self while embracing and celebrating the new. Menopause ... "the change" ... truly a gift to be welcomed.

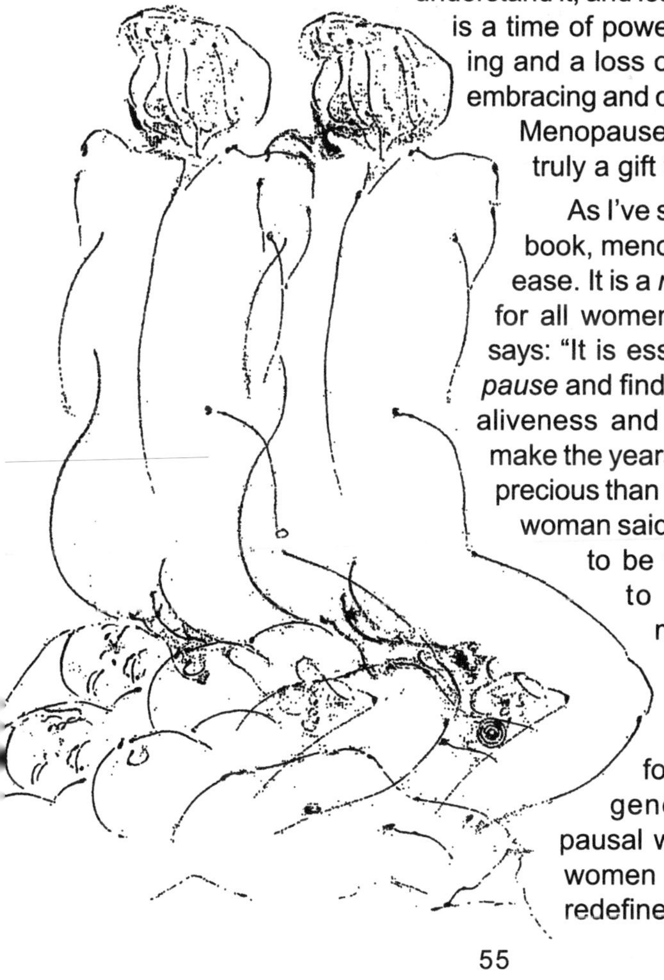

As I've said throughout this book, menopause is not a disease. It is a *normal* life transition for all women. As Gail Sheehy says: "It is essential to *claim the pause* and find this new source of aliveness and meaning that will make the years ahead even more precious than those past." As one woman said, "I don't know how to be fifty. I'm not going to be fifty like my mother, and there haven't really been any models." It *is* different for this baby boomer generation of menopausal women and for the women who follow as we redefine ourselves.

You can be a conscientious consumer of quality health care by taking charge and learning about what is happening to your body. Question your doctor. Critically read contradictory information. Gather medical histories from your family members. *Talk with other women who have been through or are going through menopause!* No one knows your body better than you, not even your doctor! You can do as your doctor tells you or research and make decisions *with* your doctor. *You can take responsibility for what happens to your body.* Yes, it's scary, but who can make a better choice than you?!

Listen to your body. What you need depends on you, your symptoms, your beliefs and how you feel. You can make choices that fit for you. You have the right to quality health care, to having a good health care provider who respects your wishes, who gives you complete information, who has a similar philosophy to yours. If you can't discuss your opinions, your feelings, and your concerns with your doctor, then you can't trust your health care to this individual. As Dr. Gary Klepper says, "Trust yourself; if something doesn't make sense to *you*, then it doesn't make sense."

In closing, I'd like to quote Rebecca Latimer's book. While she was not talking specifically about menopause, the point she makes about aging speaks to me. I hope it will speak to you as well. She says: "...I can say with all honesty, I'd rather be a very old woman than a very young one. It is true that I have lost my physical resilience, but new friends and interests outweigh my losses. Yes, I'd rather be over seventy than under fifty." Find the joy in your life. It is, after all, *your life*!

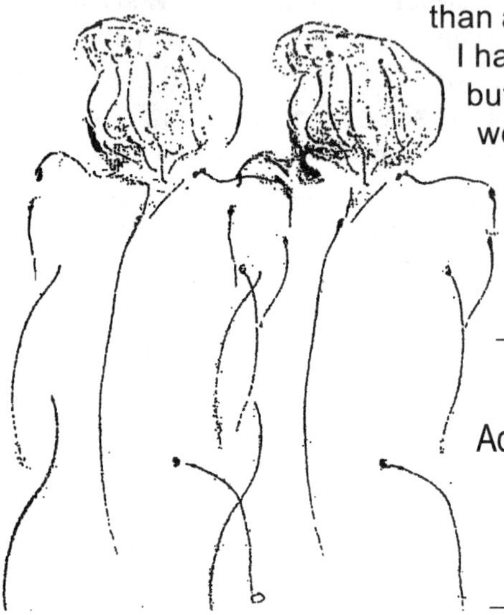

Adventure is worthwhile in itself.

Amelia Earhart

CHAPTER NINE:

For More Information

The following is a list of books and resources that I found helpful. I am not being paid by any of these individuals, businesses or organizations. I included them because I like what they are doing or found their products or books to be helpful and I wanted to share them with you. Hopefully, you will find them to be helpful too.

Resources

Aeron Laboratories can provide information about saliva hormone testing. Their automated system can be reached at 800-631-7900. They'll either send you information or you can listen to it over the phone.

Great Smokies Diagnostic Laboratories provides saliva hormone testing and bone resorption testing, among other things. Call their toll-free number: 800-522-4762.

Lois Johnson, MD, is a general practitioner and an herbalist who specializes in women's health. Her office in Sebastopol, California offers monthly classes in the use and preparation of herbs. In addition, they have an on-going group for people who want to learn more about herbs. Her office number is 707-829-8750. The herb room number is 707-824-1491.

Dr. John Lee is the author of several excellent books on menopause. These are: *Natural Progesterone, The Multiple Roles of a Remarkable Hormone* (1993), *What Your Doctor May Not Tell You About Menopause* (Warner Books, 1996), and *What Your Doctor May Not Tell You about Premenopause* (1999). His fourth book is scheduled to be released in 2000, *What Your Doctor May Not Tell You About Breast Cancer*. To purchase his books, call 800-528-0559 or www.johnleemd.com

HERS Foundation (Hysterectomy Education and Resources Services), Nora Coffey, Executive Director, is a non-profit organization that provides information and education for doctors and laypeople on alternatives to hysterectomies. This has been a very important resource for me as I watch my friends struggling through the maze of information (or lack thereof) about fibroids and endometriosis. Call them at 610-667-7757. While they do not charge a fee, I recommend sending them a donation so we can maintain this important service to women.

MoonMaid Botanicals, Cynthia Johnston, 305-253-7853, FAX: 305-253-5956,13870 SW 90th Avenue, Miami, FL 33176. All of her products are all natural (The real all natural—I can read and recognize everything that's in them!) Not only does she make Pro-Meno for menopausal symptoms, but also Radiant Rose and Dandelion face

cont. creams; Vital Vulva which helps restore the elasticity and moisture to the vagina; Yeast Free for yeast infections, Calendula Cream for dry skin, Breast Balm for painful breasts, and Ouch Ointment for injuries or burns.

Women's Health Institute Lubricating Gel, 800-537-8658, manufactured by Lake Consumer Products, Inc., Vernon Hills, IL 60061.

Annotated Bibliography

Alternative Medicine, consulting editor C. Norman Shealy, MD, Ph.D. This is an essential book for your library. It is an illustrated encyclopedia of natural healing. It lists a disorder and follows with a variety of alternative therapies including acupuncture, homeopathy, herbs, and home remedies. It is a very helpful book full of great information, even if you choose a different approach than recommended in the book. Published in 1997 by Bridgewater Book Co.

Coast Magazine, January/February 1996, *Medicine Man* by Carolyn Agosta. Published by Joy Ink, Gualala, CA.

Creative Menopause, by Farida Sharan, lists problems and possible causes as well as recommendations for treatment. Quite beautifully written. Published in 1994 by Wisdome Press, a division of the School of Natural Medicine, Boulder, Colorado.

Hormone Book, The— by Susan Love, explains menopause in great detail; thoroughly examining hormones, how they fluctuate, their affects on women, societal attitudes in this country and other countries, heart disease, osteoporosis, hormone replacement, and natural alternatives. It's the first straightforward, no-nonsense approach I have ever read. She writes a very clear and unbiased account of the benefits of hormones, the problems, what the doctors are trying to do, and the role of drug companies. If I were searching for a doctor to help me with my menopause, I'd want to know that they had read this book. And I recommend that any woman who wants to understand menopause read it as well. In addition, Dr. Love has included a list of manufactured hormones for HRT with information about the manufacturer, dosage, etc. Published in 1997 by Random House.

Menopausal Years, by Susun S. Weed describes disorders and remedies taking a natural approach to menopause. While this book is slightly older, it is still a good addition to your library. Published in 1992 by Ash Tree Publishing.

Menopause Handbook, The — by Susan Flamholtz Trien gives considerable detail about exercise, diet, hormone replacement, and potential symptoms of menopause. Very clearly written. Published in 1986 by Ballantine Books.

Menopause Industry: How the Medical Establishment Exploits Women, The—by Sandra Coney is an explosive book in which Coney explicitly tells the story of how menopause became a disease and estrogen the "modern" cure-all for women's woes. This provocative book received raves in publications including the *Washington Post*, the *San Francisco Chronicle*, and *Ms. Magazine*. It shows how menopausal myths have been built on incomplete and often misquoted research to help pharmaceutical companies and doctors sell products and services. Sandra Coney is a women's health activist and adviser to the New Zealand Minister of Health. She also wrote *Hysterectomy* and *The Unfortunate Experiment*, published by Hunter House Publishing Company, Alameda, CA in 1994.

Menopause, Naturally, by Sadja Greenwood, MD, takes a somewhat of a holistic approach to menopause. She does have a section with a self-rating scale to help women decide whether or not they should take HRT, which implies that HRT actually does make a difference. First published in 1984 by Volcano Press. (It has been revised twice.)

Menopause Self Help Book, The—by Susan M. Lark, MD, 4th edition. This book is full of menopause information from recipes and exercises to acupressure massages for all kinds of female-related discomforts. It's a must for your women's health books collection! Published 1998 by Celestial Arts.

Natural Healing in Gynecology, by Rina Nissim is a somewhat complicated, very useful reference book about women's health, disorders, and herbal treatments. While this is an older book, it has much relevant information about alternative care. Published in 1984 by Pandora.

Natural Hormone Replacement for Women Over 45, by Jonathan Wright, MD, and John Morgenthaler explains safe alternatives to traditional HRT. The authors discuss both conventional and natural treatment of menopausal symptoms while criticizing the medical profession and drug companies for their role in introducing dangerous and foreign substances into women's bodies. Published in 1997 by Smart Publications.

30 Safer Solutions for Women's Health Problems, by Adrianne Appel, *Natural Health Magazine*, April 2000, is an excellent article on alternatives to prescribing the pill for hormone-related problems. The experts for this article include Susan Lark, MD and Christiane Northrup, MD.

150 Most-Asked Questions about Menopause, by Ruth S. Jacobowitz is exactly want the title says. Its leanings are strongly toward hormone replacement rather than alternatives. Published in 1993 by Hearst Books.

The Right Dose, How to Take Vitamins & Minerals Safely, by Patricia Hausman, M.S. is a comprehensive guide about vitamins and minerals. Though published 13 years ago, it is still an excellent reference book. Published in 1987 by Rodale.

The Silent Passage: Menopause, by Gail Sheehy provides "normalcy to a normal process." Through interviews with women, with experts in the field, and her own wonderfully grounded opinion, she opens the doors to understanding what menopause is all about. Published in 1992 by G. Merritt Corporation.

Strong Women, Strong Bones: Everything You Need to Know To Prevent, Treat, and Beat Osteoporosis, by Miriam E. Nelson and Sarah Wernick (Contributor). Published by Putnam Publishing Group April 2000.

What Your Doctor May Not Tell You about Menopause, by John R. Lee, MD who is in the forefront of changing doctors' attitudes about menopause and the fallacy of estrogen deficiency. His book discusses in great detail the benefits of progesterone in its natural form particularly for osteoporosis. Additionally, he discusses research, the medical community, pharmaceutical companies' role in the training of doctors, and loads of information about balancing hormones naturally. Published in 1996 by Warner Books.

Women of the 14th Moon: Writings on Menopause, edited by Dena Taylor and Amber Coverdale Sumrall, are writings by women about their experiences with menopause. Published in 1991 by The Crossing Press.

Women's Bodies, Women's Wisdom, by Christiane Northrup, MD is all about women reclaiming our bodies. Dr. Northrop discusses the spectrum of health issues. Her book is an easy to read approach to women's health care. It is effortless reading. It's the kind of book every woman's library should have. I highlighted the book and periodically go back and reread sections. Published in 1994 by Bantam Books.

You're Not Old Until You're Ninety...Best to Be Prepared, However, by Rebecca Latimer, is an account of one woman's journey through life. It is full of wisdom, honesty, passion, and wit. It's truly a guide to living a full life, and as she says, it's never too late to change. Published in 1998 by Blue Dolphin Publishing.

The Internet as a source of information: The Internet has a wealth of information and a bunch of inaccurate junk. As you browse, find out who is producing the information. If it is a pharmaceutical company they may have ulterior motives for saying what they are. Read skeptically and *don't assume that the source is knowledgeable* simply because they are providing information. Who is providing the information, if it's free, why is it free? Are they trying to sell something? Check more than one or two sources.

CHAPTER TEN:

Glossary of Common Terms

The following list of terms is intended to provide definitions and explanations for more common terms used in discussion of the female anatomy. For more detailed information read Drs. Susan Love and Christiane Northrup.

Bartholin's Glands are two glands located on either side of the vagina secreting mucus that helps provide lubrication during sexual intercourse.

Calcitonin is a hormone produced by the parathyroid, thyroid, and thymus glands. It is responsible for increasing the amount of calcium and phosphate deposited on bones.

Climacteric is a period of decreased reproductive capacity in men and women caused by declining levels of sex hormones in the body.

Continuous combined HRT is the type of therapy for postmenopausal women who do not want to have periods.

Corpus Luteum is the remains of the follicle following ovulation. The corpus luteum secretes progesterone and is eventually resorbed by the ovary.

Cortisol is a hormone that helps to regulate many bodily functions including energy and it helps to moderate immune and inflammation responses. It is produced in the adrenal glands.

DHEA (dehydroepiandosterone) is a potent hormone that is produced by the adrenal glands. It contributes to a large portion of the body's estrogen and testosterone and to overall health and energy.

Dysmenorrhea is a medical term for menstrual cramps, effecting about 60% of the female population and probably a much higher proportion of the perimenopausal women.

Endometrium is the mucus membrane lining the uterus. It is shed with each period.

Endometriosis is a condition in which pieces of uterine tissue are present in other areas of the abdomen. This is characterized by formation of a cyst, adhesions, and menstrual pains.

Estradiol is the type of estrogen women produce before menopause. Estradiol is the most stimulating to the breast tissue.

Estrogen is a female hormone produced by the ovary and responsible for regulating certain reproductive functions. There are three types of estrogen: estradiol, estrone, and estriol. Estrogen is involved in breast development and, depending on the type of estrogen, may promote the growth of some types of breast cancer. Men have small amounts of estrogen.

Glossary cont.

Estrogen Quotient (EQ) is simply a measure of the ratio of estriol to the total of estradiol + estrogen in the urine.

Estriol is an estrogen that is produced in large amounts during pregnancy. In several studies estriol inhibited cancerous lesions of the breast, indicating that it may actually prevent cancer.

Estrone is the hormone naturally present after menopause. Estrone is believed to be more carcinogenic than estradiol.

Follicles are the eggs encased in their sacs (waiting to drop at ovulation).

Follicular Phase is the span of time between menses and ovulation.

FSH stands for **f**ollicle **s**timulating **h**ormone; it comes from the pituitary gland. FSH stimulates the follicles to produce estrogen. Estrogen rises causing the hypothalamus to secrete LH-releasing hormone that tells the pituitary to stop the FSH and produce a rush of LH.

Gonadotrophins are a collective term for follicle stimulating hormone (FSH) and luteinizing hormone (LH).

Hormone is a substance that is produced in one part of the body, passes into the bloodstream, and is carried to other organs or tissues to modify their structure or function. Hormones also help to regulate calcium metabolism.

Hysterectomy is the surgical removal of the uterus.

HRT is hormone replacement therapy – the use of synthetic hormones is in order to regulate a woman's hormone levels during one or all of the following phases: perimenopause, menopause, and post-menopause. Some of the common side effects of HRT are: fluid retention, bloating, weight gain, breast tenderness, nausea, depression not attributed to other factors, dizziness, shortness of breath, vaginal discharge, headaches and migraines, and acne. Some of the serious side effects of HRT are thromboembolic disease (body is more likely to form blood clots), endometriosis, lupus (an autoimmune disease attacking almost every organ of the body), high blood pressure, thyroid problems, fibroid tumors, ovarian cancer, gallstones, hyperplasia (extra cells form in the milk ducts of the breast), hypoglycemia (low blood sugar), asthma, melanoma, and lung cancer.

Hyperestrogenism is a condition in which a woman has too much estrogen and not enough progesterone.

LH is luteinizing hormone created in the pituitary gland. When it is at its peak in a woman's body, she ovulates. It works in conjunction with FSH.

Glossary cont.

Lumpectomy is surgery to remove only the abnormal breast tissue; it is usually followed by radiation therapy.

Mammogram is an x-ray of the breast. To prepare for the x-ray, the technician squeezes and flattens the breast between two pieces of cold metal. There is a good deal of discussion about the dangers of this diagnostic tool. A baseline mammogram at about the age of forty is important, beyond that, discuss it with your health care provider.

Mastectomy is surgery to remove the entire breast tissue.

Menopause is the cessation of menses. The average age is fifty-one.

Natural Progesterone Cream is a plant-based hormonal cream that is rarely prescribed because it is generic, cannot be patented, and many doctors don't know about it. Women have found using this cream provides tremendous relief from menopausal symptoms.

Osteoporosis is a disease that causes loss of bone mass. Bones become porous and brittle; it frequently leads to fractured spine, wrists or hips especially in women.

Osteoblasts are bone builders. Bone is in a constant state of tearing down and rebuilding.

Osteoclasts are bone dissolvers. Both this and osteoblasts are necessary for healthy bones.

Ovarian Failure is a medical term implying that egg production is the sole purpose of the ovaries and indicating that the ovaries have run out of eggs. The fact that the ovaries run out of eggs is a *normal process* in a woman's life cycle.

Ovaries are the small, oblong reproductive organs just below the Fallopian tubes on either side of the uterus that produce eggs and hormones. The female body has the most number of eggs as a 20-week old fetus, about 20 million. From that time on, she is losing eggs. This is normal. Eggs continue to diminish until about age 45–50 when they are completely gone.

Parathyroid Hormone is a hormone, synthesized and released by the parathyroid glands, that makes sure there is enough calcium for the heart and other cells.

Phytoestrogens are plant estrogens. They are interesting in that they can bind with the estrogen receptors in a woman's body and compete with natural estrogen. That is good because phytoestrogens have the ability to lower estrogen when there is a high level and raise it when it's too low. These estrogens are known as "balancers."

Glossary cont.

Pituitary gland is a small gland near the brain, between the eyes. FSH and LH, the hormones controlling ovulation, are secreted by this gland.

Polycystic Ovary Syndrome is a condition in which the ovaries develop a thickening outer wall under which many unreleased and stimulated eggs form cysts.

Postmenopause is the time after menopause, the cessation of menses.

Pregnenolone is a precursor hormone that the body converts to DHEA and progesterone.

Progesterone is a female hormone produced by the corpus luteum after ovulation. The adrenal gland produces a small amount as support for other hormones.

Progesterone Cream (topical) has few side effects associated with it, but can include skin reactions and, in a few women, sleepiness. Greater amounts of topical progesterone increase the likelihood of drowsiness and lethargy. These are minimal compared to the side effects of synthetic progesterone (see below); consequently, the natural forms of progesterone that are relatively safer are preferred by many doctors of natural medicine.

Progestin is a synthetic progesterone. Tolerated by some, it can cause many PMS-type symptoms, including headaches, irritability, breast tenderness, abdominal cramping, increased appetite, fluid retention, moodiness, and loss of libido. In addition, progestins block HDLs (the "good" cholesterol) and lower triglycerides while increasing LDL cholesterol (the "bad" cholesterol). They may also undermine the benefits of estrogen to the libido. Other side effects include bloating, breast soreness, depression, and mood swings.

Prolactin is a hormone produced by the pituitary gland. That regulates the production of progesterone by the corpus luteum and stimulates lactation of the mammary glands.

Sequential HRT is a one pill, once a day HRT treatment containing estrogen and progestin and causing regular periods.

Testosterone is a male hormone that women have in small amounts. Deficiency in women can cause hair loss, loss of bone density, and loss of libido.

Unopposed HRT is HRT treatment using estrogen only.

Vaginal atrophy is a condition causing the lining of the vagina to become dry and lose its elasticity. It is reversible using creams, hormone balancing, masturbation, and sex.

From Baby ... to Boomer ... and Beyond!

A writer for fifteen years, Carolyn Agosta is published in magazines, newspapers, and has written chapters in books. This, however, is her first book.

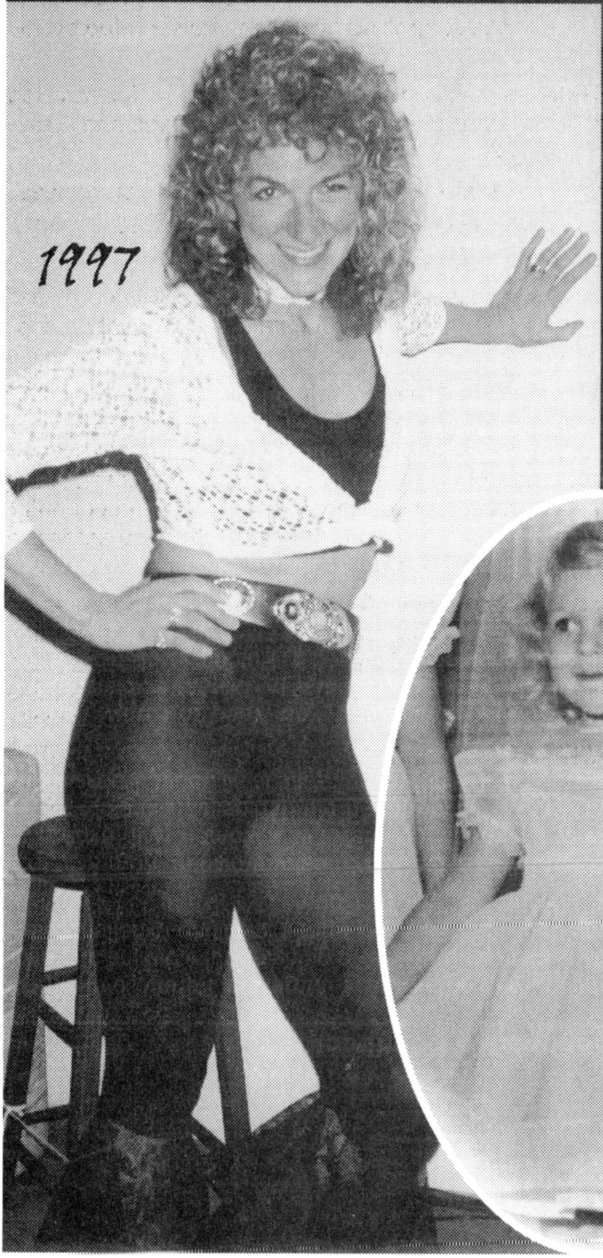

1997

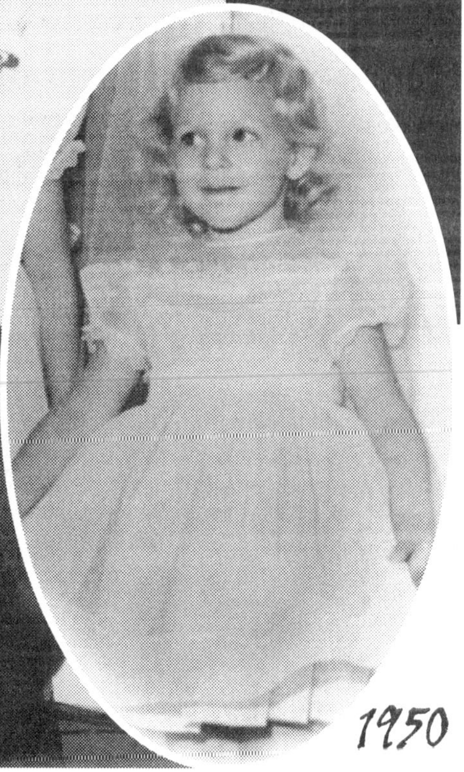

1950

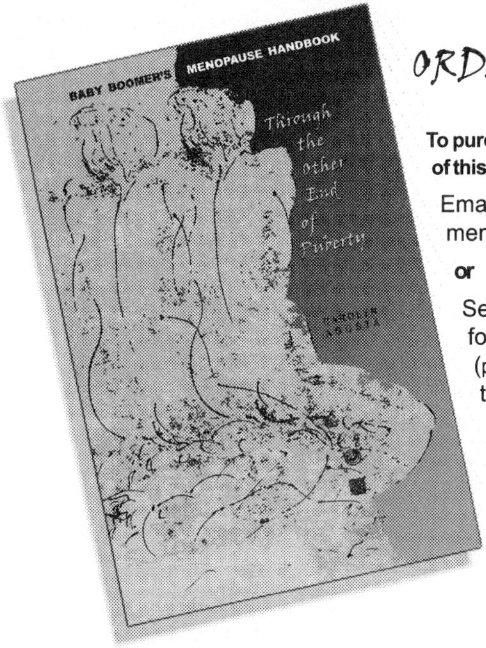

ORDER FORM

To purchase additional copies of this book:

Email CA Publishing at menopausebook.org

or

Send check or money order for $12.95
(plus $2.00 shipping)
to:
CA Publishing
35501 South Highway One
Unit 103
Gualala, CA 95445-5103
(Allow three weeks for delivery)

Use the form below, or a facsimile thereof, to place orders for **The Baby Boomers' Menopause Handbook**, *Making Your Own Choices Through the Other End of Puberty.*

Name: ____

Address: ______________________________ Apt. # ________
(P.O. Box or Street)

City: ____________________ State:_______ Zip code: ______________

Number of Books __________ x $12.95 = __________

Shipping fees: __________

Total due: __________

Shipping Fees:
1 Book ---- $2.00
2 Books --- $2.50
3 Books --- $3.00
For orders over 3 books contact publisher for special rates.